MATHEMATICS OF MICROCIRCULATION PHENOMENA

Mathematics of Microcirculation Phenomena

Editors

Joseph F. Gross, Ph.D.
Aleksander Popel, Ph.D.

*Departments of Chemical Engineering
and Physiology
University of Arizona
Tucson, Arizona*

Raven Press ■ New York

Raven Press, 1140 Avenue of Americas, New York, New York 10036

Great care has been taken to maintain the accuracy of the information contained in the volume. However, Raven Press cannot be held responsible for errors or for any consequences arising from the use of the information contained herein.

Library of Congress Cataloging in Publication Data

Symposium on Mathematics of Microcirculation
    Phenomena, Tucson, Ariz., 1979.
    Mathematics of microcirculation phenomena.

    Includes bibliographies and index.
    1. Microcirculation–Mathematical models.
2. Capillaries–Permeability–Mathematical models.
I. Gross, Joseph Francis, 1932–   II. Popel,
Aleksander. III. Title. (DNLM: 1. Microcirculation–
Congresses. 2. Mathematics–Congresses. WG104 S989m
1979)
QP106.6.S95 1979   599.01'1'072   79-5321
ISBN 0-89004-449-X

Preface

The past 2 decades have witnessed a dramatic increase in both experimental and theoretical work in microcirculatory physiology. The development of sophisticated micromeasurement techniques has made it possible to obtain data on single microvessels and this data has stimulated theoretical work whose goal is to formulate anayltical models to describe and simulate the physiological phenomena occurring in the micro-circulation. The range of mathematical approaches to the formulation of these models is broad and encompasses many methodologies.

This volume is based on presentations made at the Symposium on Mathematics of Microcirculation Phenomena, a satellite symposium of the Second World Congress for Microcirculation, held in Tucson, Arizona. The scope of the papers encompasses all of the mathematical approaches that have been employed in the solution of problems in the physiological and pharmacological phenomena in the microcirculation. The chapters are partly tutorial in that they are based on a specific mathematical approach and review the particular problem to be con-sidered. On the other hand, recent mathematical results are also included so that the contents constitute a state-of-the-art document of current developments in the modelling of microcirculatory phenomena.

This volume will be of interest to physiologists, microcirculationists, and bioengineers. It provides the life-science reader with a compendium of available mathematical methods as well as a review of the most recent models of microcirculatory physiology. The bioengineer will find a collection of analytic methods illustrating the usefulness of applications of these methods to the simulation of microcirculatory phenomena.

Joseph F. Gross, Ph.D.
Aleksander Popel, Ph.D.

Acknowledgments

The editors wish to express special thanks to Mrs. Kay Taber, administrative assistant of the Chemical Engineering Department, University of Arizona, who was conference coordinator and to Professor Paul C. Johnson, head of the Department of Physiology, for his strong support at the conference. We wish to thank the authors for providing their contributions in camera-ready format directly after the conference, and we appreciate the efforts of Larry Meyer and Nancy Derco of Raven Press for their work in the rapid publication of this volume.

Contents

Contributors

Duane Frederick Bruley. *Department of Chemical Engineering, Rose–Hulman Institute of Technology, Terre Haute, Indiana 47803*

Shu Chien. *Division of Circulatory Physiology and Biophysics, Department of Physiology, Columbia University College of Physicians and Surgeons, New York, New York 10032*

Yuan-Cheng Fung. *Department of Applied Mathematics and Engineering Sciences, University of California, San Diego, La Jolla, California 92093*

J. F. Gross. *Department of Chemical Engineering, University of Arizona, Tucson, Arizona 85721*

J. S. Lee. *Division of Biomedical Engineering, University of Virginia, Charlottesville, Virginia 22908*

H. D. Papenfuss. *Institute for Thermo and Fluid Dynamics, Ruhr-University Bochum, 4630 Bochum, Federal Republic of Germany*

Aleksander S. Popel. *Department of Physiology, College of Medicine, University of Arizona, Tucson, Arizona 85724*

Eric P. Salathé. *Center for the Application of Mathematics, Lehigh University, Bethlehem, Pennsylvania 18105*

Richard Skalak. *Department of Civil Engineering and Engineering Mechanics, Columbia University, New York, New York 10027*

Hüsnü Tözeren. *Department of Civil Engineering and Engineering Mechanics, Columbia University, New York, New York 10027*

Sheldon Weinbaum. *Department of Mechanical Engineering, The City College of The City University of New York, New York, New York 10031*

Mathematics of Microcirculation Phenomena,
edited by J. F. Gross and A. Popel.
Raven Press, New York © 1980.

Structural Mechanics of Microvasculature

Yuan-Cheng Fung

Department of Applied Mechanics and Engineering Sciences, University of California, San Diego, La Jolla, California 92093

The study of microcirculation must include the blood vessels, and the tissue surrounding blood vessels. It is well-known that blood flow and vascular elasticity are not independent of each other. Blood is driven by pressure gradient. The vessel is distended by the pressure. The pressure distribution depends on the flow and the blood vessel distension. Thus a feedback coupling exists. Normally, the elasticity of a blood vessel affects the pressure-flow relationship only in a minor way. In critical situations, however, more dramatic phenomenon can occur. For example, in a flexible vessel subjected to negative transmural pressure, the phenomenon of flow limitation may occur, at which the flow becomes independent of the venous pressure: no matter how low the venous drainage pressure is reduced to, the blood flow cannot be increased. This is aptly called the "waterfall" phenomenon, in analogy with waterfalls whose flow rate does not depend on how far the water has to plunge over the cliff. In the case of a cylindrical blood vessel, flow limitation is caused by the flow speed catching up with the speed of flexural waves in the vessel. This often happens when the blood vessel is subjected to an external pressure so high as to cause the vessel to buckle. A buckled vessel is so flexible that the wave speed can be reduced to the level of the flow speed. A "sonic" section is then created. This sonic section controls the maximum rate of flow $(\dot{Q}_{max})$ which is equal to the sound velocity (v_s) multiplied by the cross sectional area (A_s). Thus

$$\dot{Q}_{max} = A_s v_s.$$

Both A_s and v_s depend on the vessel distensibility, and the transmural pressure. Thus the elasticity of the vessel holds the key to the problem. This phenomenon occurs in large veins in the thorax and abdomen when one makes various breathing maneuvers. It occurs in trachea and bronchi when one tries strenuously to force expiration. In the lung it occurs in pulmonary microcirculation when the pressure in the venules falls below the atmospheric pressure in the alveoli.

1

Thus vascular elasticity is important to physiology. It follows that change of vascular elasticity can be important to pathology, and the measurement of the vascular elasticity is significant to diagnosis and prognosis.

In this article we consider the mechanical properties of microvasculature. Microcirculation is an old subject, but the mechanics of microcirculation was studied vigorously only in recent years. To a modern worker, it appears that much of the work has to begin from the very beginning i.e. with the determination of constitutive equations of the materials. In 1968, the author said (13 , p. 4), "To an analytical mechanicist, the most serious frustration lies in the dearth of information about the material properties, i.e. the stress-strain-history laws of living tissues. Without the constitutive law, no analysis can be done. On the other hand, without the solution of boundary value problems, the constitutive laws cannot be determined. Thus, we are in a situation in which serious analyses (usually quite difficult because of nonlinearity) have to be done for hypothetical materials, in the hope that experiments will yield the desired agreement. If no agreement is obtained, new analyses based on a different starting point would become necessary".

The course of development in the last decade or two has followed this prescription. A summary of current status is presented below.

ELASTICITY OF BLOOD VESSELS

Blood vessels are not elastic bodies in the usual sense. But when they are subjected to a cyclic loading process, the stress-strain relationship becomes definite after preconditioning. For either the loading or unloading branch, a pseudo strain energy function can be used to express the stress-strain relationship.

Although a large variety of mathematical expressions have been proposed to describe stress-strain relationship in uniaxial tests (see review in ref. (14)), for biaxial and triaxial tests there are essentially only two schools: one uses polynomials (26 , 34, 42 , 46) and the other uses exponential functions (1, 5, 6,7,14, 14, 15, 16, 23, 25, 27, 30, 31, 35, 38, 40, 41, 45). Both schools utilize strain energy functions to simplify the mathematical analysis. The arterial wall is treated as a membrane; the variation of radial stress is ignored in comparison with circumferential and longitudinal stresses $S_{\theta\theta}$, S_{zz}. Let $E_{\theta\theta}$ and E_{zz} represent the circumferential and longitudinal strains defined in the sense of Green, and let a function $\rho_o W^{(2)}$ of $E_{\theta\theta}$, E_{zz} be the strain energy per unit volume in the initial, unstressed state. The superscript (2) indicates that it is a function of two strains $E_{\theta\theta}$, E_{zz} only. Differentiation of $\rho_o W^{(2)}$ with respect to $E_{\theta\theta}$, E_{zz} yields the Kirchhoff stresses $S_{\theta\theta}$, S_{zz} respectively.

A form of $\rho_o W^{(2)}$ advocated by the polynomial school is, according to Patel and Vaishnav (34),

$$\rho_o W^{(2)} = Aa^2 + Bab + Cb^2 + Da^3 + Ea^2 b + Fab^2 + Gb^3 \qquad (1)$$

where $a = E_{\theta\theta}$, $b = E_{zz}$, and A, B, ..., G are material constants. Most other authors use exponential functions. The form we prefer is

$$\rho_o W^{(2)} = \frac{C}{2} \exp[a_1(E_{\theta\theta}^2 - E_{\theta\theta}^{*2}) + a_2(E_{zz}^2 - E_{zz}^{*2})$$
$$+ 2 a_4(E_{\theta\theta}E_{zz} - E_{\theta\theta}^* E_{zz}^*)] \qquad (2)$$

where C, a_1, a_2, a_4 are material constants, and $E_{\theta\theta}^*$, E_{zz}^* are strains corresponding to an arbitrarily selected pair of stresses $S_{\theta\theta}^*$, S_{zz}^*, (usually chosen in the physiological range). In principle, it is unnecessary to specify the starred quantities, because they can be absorbed into the constant C to yield a form

$$\rho_o W^{(2)} = \frac{C}{2} \exp[a_1 E_{\theta\theta}^2 + a_2 E_{zz}^2 + 2a_4 E_{\theta\theta}E_{zz}]. \qquad (3)$$

But in practice it is very helpful to introduce $E_{\theta\theta}^*$, E_{zz}^*: not only do they characterize the distensibility of the blood vessel, they also make the constants C, a_1, a_2, a_4 much more stable for each set of specimens.

The efficacy of these mathematical expressions has been tested by Fung, Fronek, and Patitucci (23 , 24) on two grounds: (a) their ability to fit the experimental data over full range of strains of interest, and (b) the usefulness of the parameters in distinguishing the members of a family of stress-strain curves. To obtain the needed data for evaluation they tested rabbit arteries by the television dimension analyzer method. The vessels were subjected to various combinations of axial tension and internal pressure, and the strains $E_{\theta\theta}$, E_{zz} were recorded. It was found that both expressions 1 and 2 can fit the data of any given experiment very well. If a particular specimen was tested in several different protocols, and the data from each protocol were used to determine the material constants, it was found that the standard deviations of the material constants A, B, ..., G of the polynomial strain energy function are sometimes very large compared with the mean, and some of the constants change sign in different runs of the same specimen. The variations of the constants C, a_1, a_2, a_4 of the exponential strain energy function from run to run are in general smaller than the variations of the constants A, B, ..., G of the polynomial function.

When these expressions were used to fit data from different arteries (carotid, iliac, lower and upper abdominal) of the rabbit, Fung et al (23) found that the constants C, a_1, a_2, a_4 vary systematically, whereas it is difficult to detect the trend in the constants A, B, ..., G, especially because some of them change sign from positive to negative and vice versa from one artery to another. Therefore, for the purpose of evaluating systematic changes in the mechanical properties of arteries due to some parameters (e.g. anatomical location, diet, drug, age, sex, etc.), the exponential form of strain energy function is preferred.

A similar analysis of biaxial test data of human veins was done by P. Sobin (37) and the exponential strain energy function Eq. 2 was found to apply.

The Question of Parameter Identification

The question discussed above is the question of parameter identification —— determination of physical parameters from a given set of experimental data. It should be noted that although the experimental data can be fitted accurately, the parameters themselves may not have much meaning. For example, in one exper- iment quoted in Ref. (23), (rabbit carotid artery, Exp. 71, protocol P + L), we obtained the pseudo strain energy function

$$\rho_o W^{(2)} = - 2.4385 \ a^2 - 0.3589 \ ab - 0.1982 \ b^2$$
$$+ 4.6334 \ a^3 + 3.2321 \ a^2 b + 0.3743 \ ab^2 + 0.3266 \ b^3$$

which correlates with a set of experimental data with correlation coefficients 0.971 for $S_{\theta\theta}$, and 0.878 for S_{zz}. Here $a = E_{\theta\theta}$, $b = E_{zz}$ and $\rho_o W^{(2)}$ is in units of 10 KPa. For the same arterial test specimen but in another test (Exp 71.1, protocol P), the pseudo strain energy function obtained was

$$\rho_o W^{(2)} = - 8.1954 \ a^2 + 2.5373 \ ab + 0.2633 \ b^2$$
$$+ 2.7949 \ a^3 + 11.1749 \ a^2 b - 3.0092 \ ab^2 - 0.1166 \ b^3$$

which has the correlation coefficients 0.958 for $S_{\theta\theta}$ and 0.794 for S_{zz}. It is amazing that two polynomials so disparate can represent the same artery. Although the coefficient A, B, ... are very different, the stress-strain curves are essentially identical in the experimental range. In other words, the coefficients are very sensitive to small changes in the data on stress-strain rela- tionship.

Workers in viscoelasticity and other branches of physics are familiar with this situation. Lanczos (32) gives an example in which a certain set of twenty-four decay observations was analyzed and found that it could be fitted equally well by three different expressions for x between 0 and 1:

$$f(x) = 2.202 \ e^{-4.45x} + 0.305 \ e^{-1.58 \ x}$$
$$f(x) = 0.0951 \ e^{-x} + 0.8607 \ e^{-3x} + 1.5576 \ e^{-5x}$$
$$f(x) = 0.041 \ e^{-0.5x} + 0.79 \ e^{-2.73 \ x} + 1.68 \ e^{-4.96}$$

Lanczos comments: "It would be idle to hope that some other modified mathematical procedure could give better results, since the difficulty lies not with the manner of evaluation but with the extraordinary sensitivity of the exponents and amplitudes to very small changes of the data, which no amount of least-square or other form of statistics could remedy". The same could be said of the polynomials.

In order to endow each material constants in a constitutive equation with a physical meaning, one should derive the constitutive equation from basic considerations of the anatomy, histology, material composition, and ultrastructure. Some attempts in this direction have been made for tendon and the skin on the basis of collagen and elastin fiber structures. For pulmonary capillaries Fung and Sobin (20) derived a formula for its distensibility on the basis of their structures. For lung parenchyma Fung and his associates (22 , 43 , 44) have similarly derived a constitutive equation based on structural details. For arteries and veins speculations (e.g. of Azuma and Hasegawa (2)) have not yet been reduced to a mathematical form.

Inversion of Stress-Strain Relationship

If stresses are known analytic functions of strains, one should be able to express strains as analytic functions of stresses. In linear elasticity the Hooke's law can be expressed both ways. In nonlinear elasticity, however, it is not always simple to invert a stress-strain law. For example, if the stress s is a cubic function of the strain ε :

$$s = a\varepsilon + b\varepsilon^2 + c\varepsilon^3 .$$

we know that ε cannot be expressed as a rational function of s, a, b, and c. If we think of ε, s, a, b, c as tensors, then an inversion is more difficult; in fact, unknown.

But an exponential strain energy function given in Eq 2 or 3 can be easily inverted. Such an inversion is useful whenever one wishes to calculate strains from known stresses; or when one wishes to use the complementary energy theorem in numerical analysis; or when one wishes to use the hodograph method to obtain some exact solutions; or when one wishes to use the method of stress functions which is applicable still in finite deformation, because the equations of equilibrium remain linear when expressed in terms of Cauchy stresses.

The general theory is presented by Fung (17,18). Let $\rho_o W$ be the strain energy function, $\rho_o W_c$ be the complementary energy function. Let S_{ij} and E_{ij} be the Kirchhoff stress tensor and Green's strain tensor respectively. $\rho_o W$ is a function of E_{ij} and $\rho_o W_c$ is a function of S_{ij}. Then, according to continuum mechanics (10)

$$S_{ij} = \frac{\partial \rho_o W}{\partial E_{ij}} , \qquad E_{ij} = \frac{\partial \rho_o W_c}{\partial S_{ij}} \qquad (4)$$

$$\rho_o W_c = S_{ij} E_{ij} - \rho_o W \qquad (5)$$

in which the summation convention over repeated indexes is used. The problem of inversion consists of finding $\rho_o W_c$ from $\rho_o W$ through the contact transformation given in Eqs. 4 and 5.

Let us relabel the six independent components of E_{ij} as E_1, E_2, ..., E_6, and the six independent components of stresses S_{ij} as S_1, S_2, ..., S_6. Let a square matrix $[a_{ij}]$ be symmetric and nonsingular. We define a quadratic form

$$Q = \sum_{i=1}^{6} \sum_{j=1}^{6} a_{ij} E_i E_j \qquad (6)$$

and a strain energy function

$$\rho_o W = f(Q) \qquad (7)$$

where $f(Q)$ is an analytic function of Q. Then we can invert Eq. 7 as follows:

$$S_i = \frac{\partial \rho_o W}{\partial E_i} = \frac{df}{dQ} \frac{\partial Q}{\partial E_i} = 2 \frac{df}{dQ} \sum_{j=1}^{6} a_{ij} E_j$$

a solution for E_i yields the matrix equation

$$\{E_i\} = \left(2 \frac{df}{dQ} \right)^{-1} [a_{ij}]^{-1} \{S_j\} \qquad (8)$$

A substitution into Equation 6 gives

$$Q = \left(2 \frac{df}{dQ} \right)^{-2} \{S_i\}^T [a_{ij}]^{-1} \{S_j\} \qquad (9)$$

If we define a polynomial P of stresses by

$$P = \frac{1}{4} \{S_i\}^T [a_{ij}]^{-1} \{S_j\} \qquad (10)$$

then Eq. 9 becomes

$$P = Q \left(\frac{df}{dQ} \right)^2 . \qquad (11)$$

When $f(Q)$ is given, Eq. 11 can be solved for Q as a function of P.

Now according to Eq. 5,

$$\rho_o W_c = \sum_{i=1}^{6} \frac{df}{dQ} \frac{\partial Q}{\partial E_i} E_i - \rho_o W$$

Since Q is a homogeneous function of E_i of degree 2, we know by Euler's theorem for homogeneous function that $E_i (\partial Q / \partial E_i) = 2Q$. Hence

$$\rho_o W_c = 2Q \frac{df(Q)}{dQ} - f(Q) \tag{12}$$

When the solution of Eq. 11 is substituted into the right hand side of Eq. 12, it becomes a function of P, i.e. of stresses. The inversion is thus accomplished.

    Example. Consider the strain energy function given in Eq. 3. Let

$$Q = a_1 E_1^2 + a_2 E_2^2 + 2 a_4 E_1 E_2 \tag{13}$$

Then

$$\rho_o W = f(Q) = \frac{c}{2} e^Q \tag{14}$$

and Eq. 9 is reduced to

$$Q = c^{-2} (a_1 a_2 - a_4^2)^{-1} e^{-2Q} (a_2 S_1^2 + a_1 S_2^2 - 2 a_4 S_1 S_2) \tag{15}$$

In this case,

$$P = c^{-2} (a_1 a_2 - a_4^2)^{-1} (a_2 S_1^2 + a_1 S_2^2 - 2 a_4 S_1 S_2). \tag{16}$$

and P and Q is related by the universal equation

$$Q e^{2Q} = P \tag{17}$$

which is independent of the material constants. Reading Q as a function P through Eq. 17 renders Eq. 12 a function of P. Q.E.D.

ARTERIOLES

    Peripheral arterioles are rich in smooth muscle and serves the function of controlling the blood pressure in microcirculation. These vessels are so small that experimentation is very difficult. So far data are available only with respect to change of diameter in response to changes in internal pressure. Gore (48) has presented data for arterioles in cats mesentery, and the pressure diameter relationship appears very similar to that of larger arteries. Hence it is plausible that the same strain energy function (Eq. 2) applies to arteriole.

    The response of the smooth muscles in the arterioles to changes in stretch, stress, blood pressure, oxygen, norepinephrine, or other factors is the key to the regulation of blood flow. Many experiments are being done, but many more need to be done before a constitutive equation for vascular smooth muscle can be obtained. This blank is the most important one to be filled in the future.

CAPILLARY BLOOD VESSELS

    The capillaries are the smallest blood vessels whose diameter is comparable to that of the red blood cells. Their walls are thin, and semipermeable. Mass transfer between blood and tissue takes place across their walls.

As all blood vessels, the capillaries are lined with endothelium cells. The thickness of the endothelial cell lies in the range 0.1 to 1 µm. In capillaries with inner diameter ranging from 4 to 10 µm, the endothelial cells constitute the main structure of their walls. Outside the endothelial cells is the basement membrane which has a thickness of the order of 0.01 to 0.06 um. The basement membrane is often considered as the structural underpinning of the capillaries because it contains collagen, and collagen has high electric modulus. Speidel and Lazarow (39) showed that collagenase could almost completely hydrolyse the basement membrane. Majno (33) showed that in some endothelial cells of small vessels well-formed collagen (with the typical periodicity of 640 Å) is inserted into or is closely associated with the basement membrane which, however, do not possess the 640 Å periodicity, (see Hruza, (28), and Baumgartner et al. (3)).

The chemical composition of various basement membranes in specific tissues is qualitatively similar to that of the glomerulus. These membranes are rich in hydroxyproline, hydroxylysine, and glycine, indicating their collageneous nature, but differ quantitatively in their amino acid composition and in their carbohydrate content, depending on their embryologic origin and tissue localization. In diabetes, basement membranes are thickened. Where there is chronic endothelial damage, several layers of basement membranes surrounding the small vessels can be seen.

Besides these suggestive information, we have no quantitative knowledge about the mechanical property of the basement membrane. This lack of knowledge is a major hindrance to our understanding of capillary blood vessels.

Mechanically, the most interesting characteristics of the capillaries in tissues such as the mesentery and the muscle is their rigidity — with little observable change in diameter as the transmural pressure is varied from 0 to 150 cm H_2O. In contrast, the pulmonary capillaries in the lung interalveolar septa is quite distensible — the capillary sheet thickness will double itself if the transmural pressure is increased from zero to 20 cm H_2O. The fact that the peripheral capillaries are rigid was known for some time (Baez et al. (47)). In 1964, Zweifach, while visiting Caltech, proposed this as a worthy subject for research. Fung then suggested that the capillary blood vessels appear rigid because they receive support from the surrounding tissue, in which the vessels are integrally embedded. To evaluate this hypothesis, the elasticity of the surrounding tissue was measured, and this lead to an article putting forward the concept that capillaries in connective tissues are like tunnels in a gel (Fung, Zweifach and Intaglietta, 19). Fung then reasoned that if a capillary did not receive support from surrounding tissues it should be compliant. Such a case can be found in the lung, in which the pulmonary capillaries are exposed to air. At that time, the pulmonary blood flow theory was also built on the concept of rigid capillaries (see, for example, Permutt et al (49). On the conviction that this is not the case, Fung and Sobin (20,21) measured the distensibility of the pulmonary capillary blood vessels and verified that they are quite compliant; and on that basis they put forward a theory of blood flow in the lung. Thus observations from quite different points of view were brought into harmony. Now, fourteen years later, it would be useful to review that concept.

The "Tunnel in Gel" Concept Updated

The initial evaluation of the distensibility of capillaries is based on the mechanical properties of the structural components: the endothelium, the basement membrane, and the interstitial tissue beyond the basement membrane. In the mesentery, the capillaries are embedded in connective tissue. We assume that the mechanical property of the connective tissue is the same as that of the mesentery membrane as a whole. Our 1965 experiments (19) showed that the shear modulus (G) of the mesentery increases linearly with the shear stress (τ):

$$G = \mu + C_2 \, |\tau| \tag{18}$$

where μ and C_2 are constants. In the specimens tested (with the membrane stretched to the degree usually found in in vivo observations) μ ranges from 0.21 to 1.90×10^6 dynes/cm^2, and $C_2 = 8.23 \pm 2.1$ (S.D.). Using these values, and the assumption that the endothelium and the basement membrane have a Young's modulus of the order of 10×10^6 dynes/cm^2 (similar to arteries), we analyzed the distensibility of vessels of various sizes and different thicknesses of endothelium and basement membranes centrally or eccentrically embedded in a membrane of total thickness 60 μm, (11,12). The results show that the gel outside the basement is the factor providing the major share of the rigidity of the vessel. When the vessel lumen is 5 μm, endothelium thickness is 1 μ, basement membrane 0.01 μ, then 99.7% of the capillary rigidity comes from the gel. When the vessel lumen is 12 μ, endothelium is 2 μ, basement membrane is 1 μ, then 61% of the rigidity comes from the gel.

These figures can be disputed if the Young's modulus of basement membrane is much higher (e.g., if it were the same as that of collagen, in the range of $0.1 - \times 10^9$ dyn/cm^2) or under circumstances where it is much thicker. If the basement membrane is much stiffer than either the endothelium or the gel tethering, then the pressure load will be resisted by the basement membrane.

We know little more concerning elastic modulus of the basement membrane today than in 1966, but the material properties of the connective tissue and endothelium are better understood at present. For a connective tissue subjected to plane stress, the strain energy function $\rho_0 W$ is of the form

$$\rho_0 W = C \exp \{a_1 E_{11}^2 + a_2 E_{22}^2 + a_4 E_{11} E_{22} + a_5 E_{12}^2\} \tag{19}$$

similar to Eq. 3. In the range of relatively small shear Eq. 3

is consistent with Eq. 1.

Equation 19 tells us that the connective tissue softens when the stresses in it are reduced. In the mesentery this feature is significant. It implies that if the rigidity of the mesenteric capillaries is derived from the surrounding gel, then a reduction of stresses in the mesentery will make the capillaries more distensible. At zero stress the capillaries should be quite distensible. This suggests an experimental approach to verify the tunnel-in-gel concept, although this experiment has not yet been done. Intra-vital microscopic observations of mesentery, omentum, the bat's wing, and muscles all involve a stretching out the tissue, frequently to the extent that the tensile stresses in the tissue is considerable.

On the other hand, the rigidity of endothelium is probably overestimated in our 1966 paper, in which $E = 10 \times 10^6$ dyn/cm^2 is assumed. If the protoplasm in the endothelial cells can be assumed to be a viscous fluid as in other cells (see Scott Blair (36) for a review), then the elasticity of endothelium must be derived from cell membrane. During the last 10 years the mechanical properties of red cell membranes have been clarified by Katchalsky, Evans, Hochmuth, Skalak, and others [see summary review in (8)]. The Young's modulus of the RBC membrane is of the order of 10^4 dyn/cm^2. The areal modulus (elastic modulus for change of membrane surface area per unit area) is of the order of 10^8 dyn/cm^2. If endothelial cell membrane is similar to that of the red cell membrane, then since under varying blood pressure the endothelial cell membrane can deform without changing surface area, its elastic modulus must be quite low, in the 10^4 dyn/cm^2 range. If we introduce this correction to our 1966 paper (19), then the extent of the contribution to capillary rigidity provided by the surrounding gel and the basement membrane will be increased.

In summary, depending on how rigid the basement membrane is, the percentage contribution of the surrounding gel to the vessel rigidity may vary accordingly.

In the contrasting case of the pulmonary interalveolar septa, in which the pulmonary capillaries form a sheet, the distensibility can be described by the equation (Ref. 21)

$$h = h_o + \alpha \, (p_{blood} - p_{alveoli}) \qquad (20)$$

for $p_{blood} > p_{alveoli}$, where h is the average thickness of the vascular sheet h_o is the value of h when p_{blood} tends to equal $p_{alveoli}$. If the blood pressure is smaller than alveolar gas pressure, then the capillaries buckle and $h \to 0$. If $p_{blood} - p_{alveoli}$ exceeds 20 cm H$_2$O then h tends asymptotically to a constant. α is the compliance constant. Experimental values for the cat are $h_o = 4.28$ μ, $\alpha = 0.219$ μ per cm H$_2$O, and for the dog: $h_o = 2.5$ μ, $\alpha = 0.122$ μ per cm H$_2$O. It can be shown (20) that Eq. 20 and these constants can be "explained" by the tension and curvature of the membranes and the distensibility of the "post" cells.

The pulmonary capillary sheets provide further evidence in support of the surrounding gel concept. In the plane of the interalveolar septa, all of the space surrounding the capillaries is occupied by the "posts". There is no vacant space. Therefore the capillaries and posts support each other and it is expected that they appear rigid in the plane of the interalveolar septa. Indeed, experimental observation show that the caliber of the pulmonary capillaries in the plane of the interalveolar septa is unaffected by the blood pressure, (20,21).

The distensibility of the capillaries in the skeletal muscle was observed by Fronek and Zweifach (9) who found no measurable change in capillary diameter when the capillary blood pressure was elevated up to levels as high as 40-50 mm Hg.

In liver and kidney where the interstitium is thin, and in non-mammalian species such as the frog where the connective tissue is more sparse the capillaries are expected to be more compliant than those in the mesentery: but experimental data are lacking. In the wing of the bat, Bouskela and Wiederhielm (4) recently applied external pressure to the body of the animal and observed a slow increase in diameter of some 15 to 8t percent depending on whether the capillaries are on the arterial or venous portion of the network. The pressurization of the body increases the bat's systemic blood pressure. The wing was exteriorized (stretched beyond the pressurizing box), and exposed to atmospheric pressure, so that the transmural pressure in the blood vessels was increased by the body pressurization. The bat's wing result is unique, and deserves closer investigation. It reopens the question whether there is contractile control in the capillaries.

The mechanical concept of "tunnel in gel", originally introduced as a figure of speech to explain the rigidity of the capillaries, has been extended by Intaglietta and de Plomb (29) to the fluid movement in the interstitium. In this extension the main object of interest is the assessment of the location of the hydraulic resistance to fluid movement: whether it is concentrated in the capillary wall, or is distributed in the connective tissue surrounding the capillary.

CONCLUSION

The methods of the theory of elasticity have helped us to understand the mechanical properties of the microvasculature. Yet the blood vessels and the surrounding tissues are not elastic. Their properties are history dependent. Only when the tissue is subjected to cyclic motion and preconditioned can the tissue be treated as elastic in some restricted sense. Hence we introduce the term "pseudo-elasticity" for the mathematical description of the mechanical properties of such tissues.

In microvasculature, the relationship between a blood vessel and the tissue surrounding it is important. In case of the capillaries in the mesentery and skeletal muscle, the distensibility of the vessels is largely controlled by the surrounding tissue. For the capillaries in the lung, the surrounding tissue is small

in size and insignificant in effect.   In these pulmonary capillaries it is the tension in the vessel wall that controls their
compliance with respect to transmural pressure.   These examples
illustrate the general principle that the property of a tissue
depends not only on the materials of construction, but also on
its structure, and on the stresses and strains acting in it.

The constitutive equation of the vascular smooth muscle is yet
unknown: its identification would be a worthy objective of the
next decade.

REFERENCES

1. Ayorinde, O.A., Kobayashi, A.S. and Merati, J.K. (1975):
    Finite elasticity analysis of unanesthetized and anesthetized
    aorta. In: Proceedings of Biomech. Symposium. ASME, p. 79.

2. Azuma, T. and Hasegawa, M. (1971): A rheological approach to
    the architecture of arterial walls. Japan J. Physiol. 21:27-
    47.

3. Baumgartner, H.R., Stemerman, M.B., and Spaet, T.H. (1971):
    Adhesion of blood platelets to subendothelial surface dis-
    tinct from adhesion to collagen. Experientia. 27:283-285.

4. Bouskela, E. and Wiederhielm, C.A. (1979): Microvascular
    myogenic reaction in the wing of the intact, unanesthetized
    bat. Microvascular Res. (in press).

5. Brankov, G., Rachev, A., and Stoycheve, S. (1974): On the
    mechanical behavior of blood vessels. Biomechanica.
    Bulgarian Acad. Sci. Sofia. 1:27-37.

6. Demiray, H.J. (1972): A note on the elasticity of soft
    bilogical tissues. J. Biomechanics. 5:309-311.

7. Doyle, J.M., and Dobrin, P.B. (1971): Finite deformation
    analysis of the relaxed and contracted dog carotid artery.
    Microvascular Res. 3:400-415.

8. Evans, E.A., and Skalak, R.: Mechanics and thermodynamics
    of biomembranes. Book manuscript to be published by CRC
    Press. (in press).

9. Fronek, K., and Zweifach, B.W. (1975): Microvascular pres-
    sure distribution in skeletal muscle and the effect of vaso-
    dilation. American J. of Physiol. 228:791.

10. Fung, Y.C. (1965): Foundations of Solid Mechanics.
    Prentice Hall, New Jersey.

11. Fung, Y.C., editor (1966): Microscopic blood vessels in the mesentery. In: Biomechanics. ASME. pp. 151-166.

12. Fung, Y.C. (1966): Theoretical considerations of the elasticity of red cells and small blood vessels. Federation Proceedings 25: 1761-1772.

13. Fung, Y.C. (1968): Biomechanics: Its scope, history and some problems of continuum mechanics in physiology. Applied Mechanics Reviews. 21:1-20.

14. Fung, Y.C., editor (1972): Stress-strain-history relations of soft tissues in simple elongation. In: Biomechanics: Its Foundations and Objectives. Prentice-Hall, Inc., Englewood Cliffs, New Jersey, pp. 181-208.

15. Fung, Y.C. (1973): Biorheology of soft tissues. Biorheology 10:139-155.

16. Fung, Y.C. (1975): On mathematical models of stress-strain relationship for living soft tissues. Mechanika Polymerov LSSR. 10:850:867.

17. Fung, Y.C. (1979): On pseudo-elasticity. In: Mechanics Today, Vol. IV. edited by Nemat-Nasser. Pergamon Press.

18. Fung, Y.C. (1979): Inversion of a class of nonlinear stress-strain relationships of biological soft tissues. J. Biomechanical Eng. Trans. ASME. 101(1):23-27.

19. Fung, Y.C., Zweifach, B.W., and Intaglietta, M. (1966): Elastic environment of the capillary bed. Circ. Res. 19:441-461.

20. Fung, Y.C., and Sobin, S.S. (1972): Elasticity of the pulmonary alveolar sheet. Circ. Res. 30:451-469.

21. Fung, Y.C., and Sobin, S.S. (1977): Pulmonary alveolar blood flow. In: Bioengineering Aspects of Lung Biology edited by J.B. West, pp. 267-358. Marcel Dekker, Inc. New York.

22. Fung, Y.C., Tong, T., and Patitucci, P. (1978): Stress and strain in the lung. J. Engineering Mechanics. Div. Proc. of Amer. Soc. Civil Engineering. 104(EMI): 201-223.

23. Fung, Y.C., Fronek, K., and Patitucci, P. (1979): On pseudo elasticity of arteries and the choice of its mathematical expression. American Journal of Physiol. (in press).

24. Fung, Y.C., Fronek, K., and Patitucci, P. (1979): On the choice of mathematical expressions to describe the elasticity of arteries. In: 1979 Biomechanics Symposium. American Soc. of Mech. Engineers. New York. AMD Vol. 32. pp. 115-118.

25. Gou, P.E. (1970): Strain energy function for biological tissues. J. Biomechanics. 3:547-550.

26. Greenfield, J.C., and Patel, D.J. (1962): Relation between pressure and diameter in the ascending aorta of man. Circ. Res. 10:778-781.

27. Hayashi, K., Sato, M., Handa, H., and Moritake, K. (1974): Biomechanical study of the constitutive laws of vascular walls. Experimental Mechanics. 14:440-444.

28. Hruza, Z. (1977): Connective tissue. In: Microcirculation, Vol. 1, edited by G. Kaley and B.M. Altura., Ch. 7, pp. 167-183, Univ. Park Press, Baltimore.

29. Intaglietta, M., and de Plomb, E. (1973): Fluid exchange in tunnel and tube capillaries. Microvascular Res. 6:153-168.

30. Kasyanov, V. (1974): The anisotropic nonlinear model of human large blood vessels. Mechanical Polymerov, USSR. 874-884.

31. Kasyanov, V., and Knets, I. (1974): Strain energy function for large human blood vessels. Mechanica Polymerov. USSR. 122-128.

32. Lanczos, C. (1956): Applied Analysis. p. 276. Prentice-Hall, Inc., Englewood Cliffs, New Jersey.

33. Majno, G. (1965): Ultrastructure of the vascular membrane. In: Handbook of Physiology, Sec. 2, Vol. 2. Edited by H. Hamilton and P. Dow. pp. 2293-2375. American Physiological Society, Washington, D.C.

34. Patel, D.J., and Vaishnav, R.N. (1972): The rheology of large blood vessels. In: Cardiovascular Fluid Dynamics, edited by D.H. Bergel., Vol. 2, Chap. 11, pp. 2-65. Academic Press, New York.

35. Purina, B.G., Vilka, Y., Kasyanov, V., and Ceders, E. (1974): Change of some mechanical properties of human large blood vessels with age. Mechanica Polymerov, USSR, 129-138.

36. Scott Blair, G.W. (1974): <u>An Introduction to Biorheology</u>. Elsevier Co., New York.

37. Sobin, P. (1977): Mechanical properties of human veins. M.S. Thesis, AMES-Bioengineering Department, at University of Calif., San Diego.

38. Snyder, R.W. (1972): Large deformation of isotropic biological tissue. <u>J. Biomechanics</u>. 5:601-606.

39. Speidel, E., and Lazarow, A. (1963): Chemical composition of glomecular basement membrane material in diabetes. <u>Diabetes</u>. 12:355.

40. Tanaka, T.T., and Fung, Y.C. (1974): Elastic and inelastic properties of the canine aorta and their variation along the aortic tree. <u>J. Biomechanics</u>. 7:357-370.

41. Tong, P. and Fung, Y.C. (1976): The stress-strain relationship for the skin. <u>J. Biomechanics</u>. 9:649-657.

42. Vaishnav, R.N., Young, J.T., Janicki, J.S. and Patel, D.J. (1972): Nonlinear anisotropic elastic properties of the canine aorta. <u>Biophysical J.</u> 12:1008-1027.

43. Vawter, D.L., Fung, Y.C., and West, J.B. (1978): Elasticity of excised dog lung parenchyma. <u>J. Appl. Physiol</u>. 45:261-269.

44. Vawter, D.L., Fung, Y.C., and West, J.B. (1979): Constitutive equation of lung tissue elasticity. <u>J. Biomech. Engineering. Trans. of ASME</u> 101(1):38-45.

45. Vito, R. (1973): A note on arterial elasticity. <u>J. Biomechanics</u>. 6:561-564.

46. Wesley, R.L.R., Vaishnav, R.N., Fuchs, J.C.A., Patel, D.J., and Greenfield, Jr., J.C. (1975): Static linear and nonlinear elastic properties of normal and arterialized venous tissue in dog and man. <u>Circulation Res</u>. 37:509-520.

47. Baez, S., Lamport, H. and Baez, A. (1960): Pressure effects in living microscopic vessels. In: <u>Flow Properties of Blood and Other Biological System</u>. Edited by A.L. Copley and G. Stainsby. pp. 122-136. Pergamon Press, Oxford.

48. Gore, R.W. (1974): Pressures in cat mesenteric arterioles and capillaries during changes in systemic arterial blood pressure. <u>Circ. Res</u>. 34:581-591.

49. Permutt, S., Caldini, P., Maseri, A., Palmer, W.H.,
     Sasamori, T., and Zierler, K. (1969): Recruitment versus
     distensibility in the pulmonary vascular bed. In: The
     Pulmonary Circulation and Interstitial Space. Edited by
     A.P. Fishman and H.H. Hecht. Chicago, University of
     Chicago Press. pp. 375-387.

Mathematics of Microcirculation Phenomena,
edited by J. F. Gross and A. Popel.
Raven Press, New York © 1980.

Flow Mechanics in the Microcirculation

Richard Skalak and Hüsnü Tözeren

*Department of Civil Engineering and Engineering Mechanics, Columbia University,
New York, New York 10027*

INTRODUCTION

Through a combination of experimental results and theoretical considerations, the mechanics of flow in the microcirculation is quite well understood in both capillary blood vessels and the larger vessels of the microcirculation. However, in regard to the mathematics involved, exact analytic or even numerical solutions are scarce because of the difficulty of the problem particularly in the larger vessels, say greater than 10 or 12 microns in diameter. This is because in the larger vessels the blood cells may pass each other or flow side by side requiring for a mathematical solution the treatment of several particles at the same time. The analytical results are limited to cases in which one particle occupies a given section of the tube at a given time. Further, these solutions are carried out primarily for axisymmetric cases. This is the case to which the present paper will be primarily directed.

In capillary flow there is an interesting mechanics in which the pressure drop driving the particle is opposed by shear stresses on the particle in the region closest to the tube wall and by the resultant of pressures in this zone. The latter may be quite important. If the particle is deformable, there is a further interaction of deformation of the particle, the stress distribution on it, and the driving pressure gradient. The two cases of rigid and flexible particles will both be treated below.

There have been several reviews previously in this field and the present paper is a summary and updating of the literature. (See Skalak [18]; Goldsmith and Skalak [12]; Chien et al [7]; Sutera [21]).

GENERAL EQUATIONS

The flow in capillary blood vessels takes place at very low Reynolds number (less than 0.01). The plasma in which the blood cells are suspended is known to be a Newtonian fluid of viscosity about 1.2 centipoise. The motion of the suspending plasma may be regarded as a Stokes flow for which the equations of motion reduce to:

$$0 = -\nabla p + \mu \nabla^2 \underline{u} \tag{1}$$

where $\underline{u}$ is the vector velocity and p is the pressure. The flow must also satisfy the equation of conservation of mass:

$$\underline{\nabla} \cdot \underline{u} = 0 \tag{2}$$

The boundary conditions for the fluid motion may be taken to be zero velocity at the tube wall, matching the particle velocity and traction on the surface of suspended particles, and a specification of either the total discharge or the pressure drop over some appropriate length of the capillary. In most of the cases solved, the particles are assumed to undergo only a uniform translation. This will be the case when an axisymmetric particle is located on the axis of the capillary. This appears to occur at least approximately in some cases and allows a mathematical discussion to be evaluated in detail.

In any case, because of the low Reynolds number and small particles involved, the inertia of the particles is also negligible. Therefore, for neutrally bouyant particles, the net force on any particle and the net moment must be equal to zero. This is an important condition of the suspension flow and is called the zero drag condition. As will be explained in a later section, some of the theories given previously (Lighthill [16]; Fitz-Gerald [10]) contained an error in this regard which leads to important numerical differences. In the case of axisymmetric particles, the zero moment condition is automatically satisfied, but in the case of particles off-center, the zero moment condition is used to determine the angular velocity at which the particle will rotate (Bungay and Brenner [5]).

For deformable particles, equations of motion and appropriate constitutive equations must be satisfied also. The internal velocity and stress fields must match the fluid stresses on the boundary of the particle. These stresses depend on the particle deformation so the entire coupled problem must be solved

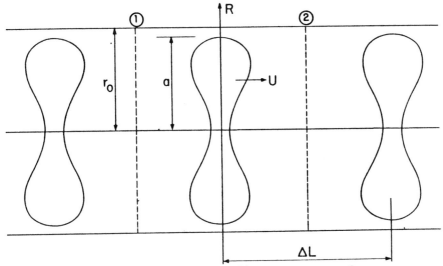

FIG. 1.   Geometry and coordinate system for a
line or particle shaped like red cells axisymmetrically situated in a circular tube containing
a Newtonian fluid.

simultaneously.   For large deformations, the problem is
highly nonlinear.

The red blood is realistically modeled as a thin,
elastic or viscoelastic shell filled with a viscous
fluid which is a hemoglobin solution of viscosity about
6 cp.   Simplified models of various types have been
used to facilitate analysis.   Lighthill and Fitz-
Gerald ([16], [10]) introduced a locally elastic cell,
in which the elastic radial compression at any point
was assumed proportional to the pressure at that point.
Hyman et al [14] used a viscous liquid droplet with
surface tension to represent the membrane elasticity.
These crude models give qualitatively correct results,
but are not accurate quantitatively or in details of
shapes or stress distributions.

RIGID PARTICLES

In a steady axisymmetric flow, solutions have been
developed for lines of spheres (Wang and Skalak [26];
Hochmuth and Sutera [13];   Bungay and Brenner [5]),
spheroids (Chen and Skalak [6]), discs (Puglierello
and Hsiao [4];   Lew and Fung [15];   Aroesty and Gross
[1]) and for biconcave rigid disc shapes (Skalak et al
[19]).   These solutions for rigid particles demonstrate

certain properties of supsension flow which do not depend strongly on the particle shape.

The first property of such flows which occurs for all of the shapes mentioned is that a particle on the axis of the capillary travels faster than the mean flow. Secondly, the pressure drop depends most strongly on the ratio of the maximum diameter of the particle to the tube diameter. This is called the diameter ratio λ which is equal to a/r_0 where a and r_0 are the maximum particle radius and tube radius, as in Fig. 1.

A third property which is common to particles of any shape is that the pressure drop due to any given particle is independent of the presence of other particles if the spacing is greater than about one tube diameter. In this case, the velocity profile approaches the parabolic Poiseuille flow between two particles. The apparent viscosity due to a suspension flow in a capillary at low hematocrits is therefore proportional to the hematocrit as shown in Fig. 2 which is computed for a line of rigid particles of red cell shape shown in Fig. 1.

When the particle spacing becomes small, there is an essentially rigid body motion of the fluid between adjacent particles. This trapping of the fluid between particles results in the surprising phenomenon that the apparent viscosity is relatively independent of hematocrit. This may be seen in the curve for $\lambda = 0.8$ in Fig. 2 in hematocrit range between 30 and 50 percent. In most cases the apparent viscosity increases with hematocrit because the diameter ratio λ will generally be greater than 0.8 in the capillaries.

The solutions graphed in Fig. 2 were obtained by a finite element method. Solutions for the case of spheres and spheroids have been previously obtained by infinite series (Wang and Skalak [26]; Chen and Skalak [6]). Such infinite series typically converge slowly when the diameter ratio λ is 0.90 or greater. For $\lambda > 0.95$, series solutions are impractical. For closely fitting particles ($\lambda > 0.95$) it is sufficient to use the lubrication theory approximations suggested by Lighthill [16]. Bungay and Brenner [5] showed that the leading term in the asymptotic expansion of pressure drop in terms of minimum gap thickness is correctly predicted by lubrication theory.

Bungay and Brenner [5] have treated an eccentrically located sphere by asymptotic expansions in which case the sphere rotates as it translates down the capillary. It is shown that in the absence of inertial effects, a neutrally bouyant homogeneous rigid sphere will move along a line parallel to the axis of the tube. Radial migration may occur if the particle is flexible [11] or if the inertial terms are taken into account at higher

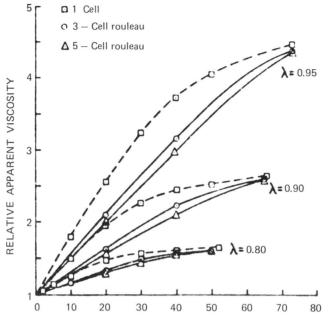

FIG. 2.   Relative apparent viscosity η_r for a
train of equally spaced single biconcave cells
(dashed curves) and reouleaux of three and five
cells respectively (solid lines) as a function
of hematocrit and diameter ratio λ (After Skalak
et al [19]).

Reynolds numbers [27].

STEADY FLOW CF SOLID ELASTIC SPHERES

The steady flow of elastic spheres in circular cylindrical tubes were considered by Tözeren and Skalak
[23],[24] using a series expansion of the particle displacements and lubrication theory for the fluid motion.
The coupled equations for the fluid and solid are
solved by an iterative numerical procedure. The results may be regarded as an approximate model of white
blood cells in capillaries although white blood cells
are known to be viscoelastic.
    Fig. 3 shows the relative apparent viscosity $\eta =
\Delta p/(16 \mu V a/r_0^2)$ computed for a line of elastic spheres
just touching each other as a function of velocity parameter $A = \mu U a/G r_0^2$ (G = shear modulus, a = particle radius, r_0 = tube radius, U = particle velocity) and initial diameter ratio $\lambda_i = a/r_0$. The value of η decreases as A increases due to substantial particle de-

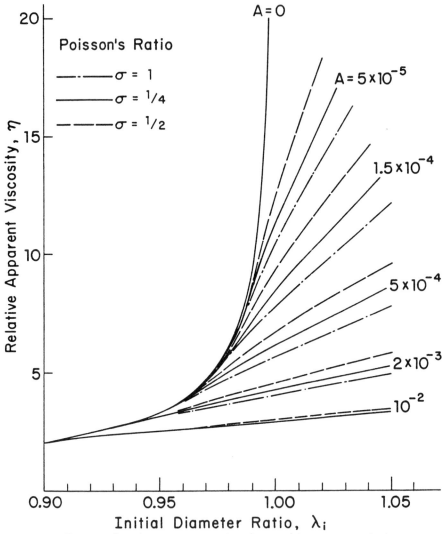

FIG. 3.   Relative apparent viscosity η vs. initial diameter ratio λ_i for various values of velocity parameter A and Poisson's ratio σ.   The
spacing between centers of spheres is one particle diameter.

formations at high velocities (or for softer particles)
for fixed values of λ_i.
    The differences between A = constant curves increase
as λ_i increases.   This is due to the decrease of fluid-
film thicknesses (which are much smaller than the elastic deformations) at greater values of λ_i.

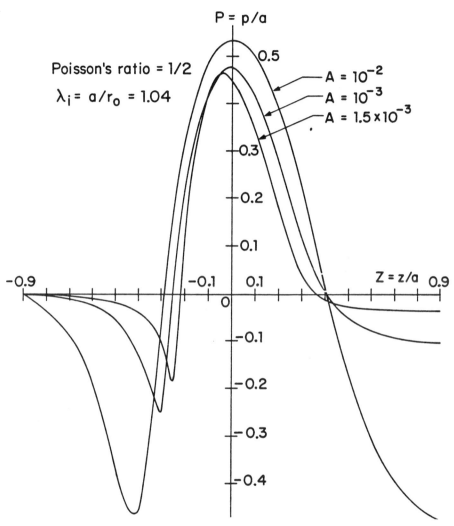

FIG. 4. Dimensionless pressure curves for deformable spheres as a function of axial coordinate and velocity parameter A for λ_i = 1.04, $\sigma = \frac{1}{2}$.

For fixed A and λ_i, the values of η decrease slightly as Poisson's ratio σ decreases from $\frac{1}{2}$ to 0 as shown in Fig. 3. However, it appears that the behavior of these curves is primarily dependent on Young's modulus E, but not on σ (Tözeren and Skalak [24]). Fig. 4 shows some typical pressures developed in the

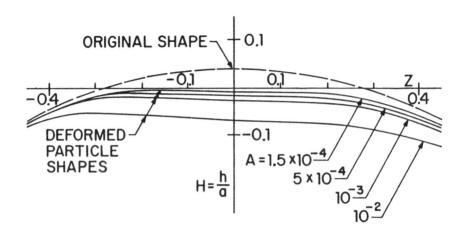

FIG. 5.   The dimensionless gap thickness for
elastic spheres as a function of axial coordinate and velocity parameter A for λ_i = 1.04
and σ = ½.

lubrication film as a function of axial coordinate
(z = 0 at the center of the particle) for fixed λ_i =
1.04 and for different values of velocity parameter A.
As A decreases, there is a substantial decrease in the
pressure drop and the negative stresses (reduced pressure region upstream of the narrowest gap).   However,
the pressures at the central region are not strongly
dependent on U or Δp as can be seen from this figure.
The reason is that when the fluid film thickness is
small compared to particle deformations, the elastic
deformations are approximately determined by the initial particle-tube geometry as described by λ_i.   The
stresses primarily responsible for producing these deformations are the central pressures.   Therefore, these
pressures are less sensitive to particle velocity or
pressure drop, but essentially determined by the initial particle-tube geometry and the elastic properties
of the particles.
   Typical particle deformations and gap thicknesses
are shown in Fig. 5.   In all the cases the particle is
incompressible and λ_i is equal to 1.04.   The film
thickness h attains its minimum on the upstream side
of the particle.   The gap can be approximated very
accurately by a straight line in the central region
where build-up of lubrication pressures takes place.
As A varies between 10^{-2} and 10^{-4} the pressures in the

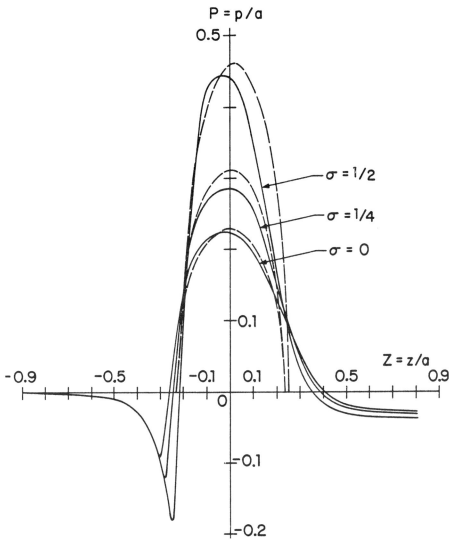

FIG. 6. Comparison of lubrication pressures for $\sigma = 0$, ¼, ½ and $A = 1.5 \times 10^{-4}$, $\lambda_i = 1.04$ with elastic contact pressures for elastic spheres.

central region do not vary appreciably because the pressures are proportional to $1/h^2$. The shear stress is proportional to A and $1/h$ so its magnitude is substantially decreased as A decreases.

The numerical results presented in Fig. 4 indicate that the pressures in a central region approach a limiting pressure distribution as $\Delta p \to 0$. In Fig. 6 the

lubrication pressures for λ_i = 1.04, A = 1.5 x 10^{-4} and
σ = 0, ¼ and ½ are compared with approximate contact
pressures which would be developed if the elastic particle is forced into a smaller tube (λ_i = 1.04) with no
lubricant present but with zero friction between the
particle and the tube. When $\lambda_i = a/r_0$ is slightly
greater than unity (contact length is small), the axi-
symmetrical contact problem for a spherical particle
and a cylindrical tube may be approximated by the contact of an infinitely elastic cylinder with a rigid
flat plane. In this case the pressures in the contact
region will have an elliptical distribution and the
maximum pressure q will be given by q = G b/r_0 (1 - σ)
where b is the half-width of the surface of contact
(Timoshenko and Goodier [22], pp. 381). This is the
basis of Fig. 6.
    Although the contact pressures shown are only an ap-
proximation to the pressures that would develop due to
the interaction of the particle with the tube in the
absence of the fluid, there is a good agreement between
the lubrication and contact pressures. This indicates
that when the thickness of the fluid film is small compared to particle deformations (U and Δp are small) the
lubrication pressures approach to the contact pressures
of the purely solid contact problem.
    Tözeren and Skalak [24] compared the results of
elastic compressible particles with the results of
Lighthill- Fitz-Gerald model. In their model, the mean
pressure may always be adjusted so that the particle,
when at rest under zero pressure drop, just fills the
capillary. Elastic incompressible particles are not
comparable with the Lighthill - Fitz-Gerald model because no reference pressure as they define it exists
for incompressible particles. The results for compressible elastic particles and the corrected Lighthill
- Fitz-Gerald theory are of similar order of magnitude
when similar parameter values are used. However, for
elastic particles the dependence of relative apparent
viscosity to initial diameter ratio is qualitatively
different than predicted by the Lighthill - Fitz-Gerald
model. The reason is that the linear local elastic
relationship used by Lighthill and Fitz-Gerald between
the pressures and displacements is not a good approximation to elastic particles even in the vicinity of the
point where film thickness attains its minimum.
    The Lighthill - Fitz-Gerald results as originally
published contains errors which make direct comparison
difficult. The principal error was in the zero drag
condition. The force on the particle due to the pressure drop was equated to the resultant of shear
stresses exerted on the particle. This omits the resultant of the lubrication pressures on the particle,

which as shown in Fig. 4, may be much larger than the applied pressures. Omission of the lubrication pressures acting on the particle can result in substantial errors. If the force balance is carried out for the fluid bounded by the tube walls and sections perpendicular to the tube axis, the lubrication pressures do not come into play because the normal to the tube wall is perpendicular to the axial direction.

FLOW OF ELASTIC SPHERES IN TAPERED TUBES

The unsteady flow of closely-fitting elastic spheres rigid truncated cones and spherical particles are considered by Tözeren and Skalak [25] under lubrication theory assumptions. Closed form solutions are found for rigid particles. In the case of elastic particles, a numerical procedure is applied to solve the equations in the fluid and the solid.

The dimensionless pressure drop $\Delta p' = \Delta p/(16\mu Va/r_0^2)$ (Δp = pressure drop across one particle, V = average velocity) as a function of λ_i, $\overline{\Delta p} = \Delta p/G$ and $\alpha = 0$, 1° and 3° is shown in Fig. 7. The differences between $\Delta p'$ curves for different values of α are small for large $\overline{\Delta p}$. These differences are greatest for rigid spheres. For rigid spheres, at the particle surface there is a velocity component in the direction of normal to the tube of magnitude U tan α where U is the particle velocity. The normal component of velocity causes substantial increases in lubrication pressures by squeeze-film action which becomes increasingly important as α increases. The resultant of these pressures in axial direction must be overcome by an increase of Δp to satisfy the equilibrium of the particle. Therefore $\Delta p'$, which is proportional to Δp, increases as α increases for fixed $\overline{\Delta p}$ and λ_i. For elastic particles, the time derivative of h (h = fluid film thickness) is smaller than U tan α because of particle deformations at its surface. Therefore, the differences between $\Delta p'$ curves for different values of α when $\overline{\Delta p}$ and λ_i are fixed are smaller than for rigid particles.

When h is small compared to elastic displacements, the pressures cannot vary significantly with α from considerations involving elasticity alone. The minimum and maximum lubrication pressures increase slightly with increasing α ($\overline{\Delta p}$, λ_i fixed); otherwise, the pressure curves are similar and close to each other (See Tözeren and Skalak [25], Fig. 6). This is in contrast with the pressure curves for rigid particles. In this case, there is a substantial increase of pressures with increasing α due to the squeeze-film motion (See Fig. 4, Tözeren and Skalak [25]).

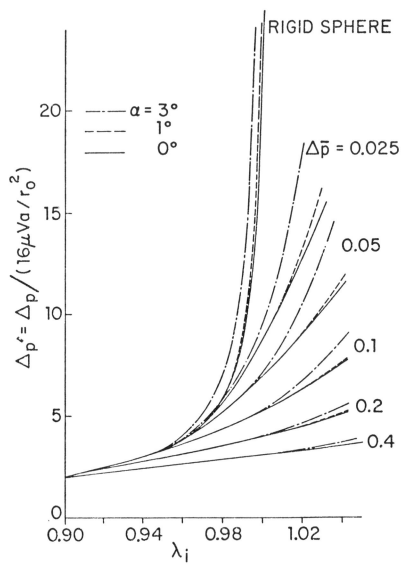

FIG. 7. The dimensionless pressure drop Δp' vs.
initial diameter ratio λ_i for various values of
$\bar{\Delta p}$ = p/a and taper angle = 0, 1° and 3° for
elastic spheres.

The numerical results also indicate that, for $\bar{\Delta p}$
fixed and for non-zero α values, the particle velocity
U approaches to zero at some limiting diameter ratio λ_i
(i.e., at a certain position along the axis of the

tube).. The numerical procedures used cannot be suc-
cessfully applied in cases involving very small gap
thicknesses. Therefore, it was not possible to inves-
tigate numerically the limiting situations involving
very small values of U. However, the contact theory
equations may be used to approximate these cases qualitatively. When h is small and α is small but non-
zero, there are basically two forces keeping the particle in equilibrium: (i) the force due to pressure
drop and (ii) the resultant in axial direction of lubrication pressures acting in a central region. By
using contact theory equations, the resultant of pres-
sures can be approximated as $P = \pi^2 G b^2 \sin \alpha / (1 - \sigma)$,
where b is the half-contact width. Equating P to the
force due to pressure drop, yields:

$$\Delta p = \frac{\pi G}{(1-\sigma)} \ (\lambda_i^2 - 1) \sin \alpha \qquad (3)$$

An elastic sphere under the application of a fixed Δp
cannot be forced further into the taper tube than $\lambda_i = a/r_0$ when there is no friction between the particle
and the tube. This limiting λ_i can be obtained from
Eq. (3) above.

For the case of particles which are rigid truncated
cones of the same angle α as the tapered tube, it is
found that the pressure has a parabolic distribution
when α is small. In this case, the maximum pressure,
p_{max} and the pressure drop, Δp are given by

$$p_{max} = \frac{-3}{2} \frac{\mu \dot{h}}{h^3} L^2, \quad \Delta p = -2 \frac{\mu \dot{h}}{h^3} \frac{L^3}{r_0} \sin\alpha \qquad (4)$$

where h is the constant gap width and $\dot{h}$ is the time
rate of change of h, L is particle length and r_0 is
the tube radius measured at the center of the particle.

For rigid spheres similar formulae are obtained
(Tözeren and Skalak [25]):

$$p_{max} = \frac{-6\mu a \dot{h}_0}{h_0^2}, \quad \Delta p = - \frac{6\sqrt{2} \ \pi \mu \dot{h}_0}{h_0^{3/2}} \ (\frac{a}{r_0})^{3/2} \ r_0^{\frac{1}{2}} \sin \alpha \qquad (5)$$

where h_0 is the minimum film thickness.

In the case of rigid particles $\dot{h} = U \sin \alpha$ (or $\dot{h}_0 = U \sin \alpha$). Then h and U may be found as a function of
time by integrating Eqs. (4) or (5) for fixed Δp. For
the elastic particles when grossly deformed into the
approximate truncated cone shape, these formulae may
again be used to determine h as a function of t and material properties. For example, for a given b (half-

contact width) the maximum contact pressure q is $Gb/r_0(1-\sigma)$. Equating q to p_{max}, L to 2b and integrating Eq. (4):

$$\frac{\dot{h}}{h} = -\frac{G}{6br_0\mu(1-\sigma)} \tag{6}$$

and

$$h = \frac{G}{3br_0\mu(1-\sigma)} (t + t_0)^{-\frac{1}{2}} \tag{7}$$

As mentioned above for rigid particles, $\dot{h}$ is equal to U sin α. However, flexible particles when sufficiently slowed down may expand to attain their limiting deformed configuration. Hence, in these cases integration of (4) or (5) may not be sufficient to obtain translational velocity U. The cases of viscoelastic particles which are better models of white blood cells (see Bagge et al [2]) are further complicated by relaxation of particles under constant stress which makes the limiting configuration a time-dependent variable.

FLEXIBLE RED BLOOD CELL MODELS

A realistic model of the red blood cell may be comprised of an elastic membrane filled with a viscous fluid. The properties of red blood cell membranes have been fairly well established by a number of different types of tests. The general picture that develops is that the red blood cell is readily deformed in the sense of changing its proportions, but is not readily changed in its surface area. It also has a bending resistance which is important to producing the smooth shape usually observed in normal red cells at rest or under moderate stresses.

The behavior of the red blood cell membrane has been established as being viscoelastic (Chien et al [8]). However, for steady flow, the elasticity of the membrane is the only property that needs to be taken into account because the cell shape does not vary with time. The elastic stresses may be defined in terms of strain energy functions. For the stresses in the plane of the membrane, the strain energy has been suggested to be of the form (Skalak et al [20]):

$$W_m = \frac{P}{4}(\tfrac{1}{2}I_1^2 + I_1 - I_2) + \frac{C}{8} I_2^2 \tag{8}$$

In Eq. (i), I_1 and I_2 are the variants of the Green's

strain tensor. They are conveniently expressed in the form:

$$I_1 = \lambda_1^2 + \lambda_2^2 - 1 \qquad (9)$$

$$I_2 = \lambda_1^2 \lambda_2^2 - 1 \qquad (10)$$

where λ_1 and λ_2 are the principal extension ratios. The coefficients B and C are elastic moduli. The coefficient B is of the order of 0.005 dyn/cm and C is of the order of 450 dyn/cm. The coefficient B controls the shear deformation and is relatively small. The coefficient C determines the areal modulus which is comparatively large. For most purposes the red blood cell membrane may be assumed to have constant area which corresponds to C approaching infinity. In this case, the term in C may be omitted and its effect replaced by a uniform isotropic tension T_0 instead. The stresses are given in terms of the strain energy by

$$T_1 = \frac{\lambda_1 B}{2\lambda_2} (\lambda_1^2 - 1) + T_0$$

$$T_2 = \frac{\lambda_2 B}{2\lambda_1} (\lambda_2^2 - 1) + T_0$$

$$(11)$$

The bending strain energy is assumed to depend on the changes of the principal curvatures. A suggested form (Zarda et al [28]) is

$$W_B = \frac{D}{2} (K_1^2 + 2\nu K_1 K_2 + K_2^2) \qquad (12)$$

In this form of the strain energy the changes of the curvature K_1 and K_2 are defined by

$$K_1 = \frac{d\theta}{\overset{\circ}{ds}} - \frac{d\overset{\circ}{\theta}}{\overset{\circ}{ds}} \qquad K_2 = \frac{\sin \theta}{\overset{\circ}{r}} - \frac{\sin \overset{\circ}{\theta}}{\overset{\circ}{r}} \qquad (13)$$

where the index ° refers to initial coordinates and the variables r and z are the radial and axial coordinates and θ is the angle of the normal with respect to the direction.

The above model has been used to compute the deformation and apparent viscosity of a line of red blood cells starting from axial position such as shown in Fig. 1 (Zarda et al [28]). This treatment starts with a variational principle of the following form

$$\delta D_m = 0 \qquad (14)$$

where D_m is a modified dissipation function which takes the form

$$D_m[\bar{u},p,T] = 2\mu \int_{V_f} e_{ij}^2 dV - 2\int_{V_f} p\theta dV - 2\int_S \underline{t}_n \cdot \underline{u} dA$$

$$+ 2\int_A T \frac{1}{\lambda_1 \lambda_2} \dot{\overline{\lambda_1 \lambda_2}} dA + 2\int_{A_o} \dot{W}_m d\mathring{A} + 2\int_{A_o} \dot{W}_B d\mathring{A} \qquad (15)$$

where the dot over the membrane strain energy and the bending strain energy indicate time rates of change, p is the pressure, θ is the rate of dilatation equal to $u_{i,i}$. It can be shown that when the functional D_m is stationary, all of the governing equations both in the fluid and solid with appropriate boundary conditions and compatibility of displacements and stresses are satisfied. The variational principle is implemented by a finite element method. The nodal variables are the radial axial velocities and the pressure at each node of the finite element network. The numerical work proceeds in two stages. For any assumed position of the red blood cell it is possible to solve for all of the fluid velocities and pressures including the velocities of the nodes on the membrane. The solution which is sought for steady flow is one in which all nodal points on the cell membrane move at the same velocity. If this condition is not satisfied the position of the membrane is adjusted until it is satisfied. At the same time the zero drag condition is incorporated into the computation.

Some results of the numerical computations are shown in Fig. 8. The hematocrit is approximately 26% in each case. In Fig. 8 the initial diameter ratio is 0.95 and the successive shapes of the particles shown are for increasing dimensionless pressure drop as indicated in the figure. In Fig. 9 a similar set of computed shapes is shown for an initial diameter ratio of 1.05. In this case there is a limit to the solutions which can be computed numerically at low pressure drops. When the particle approaches the tube wall closely, the numerical procedures become unstable because the cell tends to move beyond the tube wall which is not permissible. This is a problem of the accuracy with which the computations are carried out rather than intrinsic difficulties of the method.

Fig. 10 shows the apparent viscosities computed for several initial diameter ratios. These all represent results at approximately 26% hematocrit and assuming the cells are always axisymmetrically oriented. The fact that both the front and rear faces of the cell

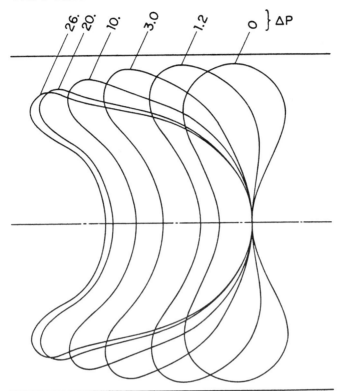

FIG. 8. Shapes computed for red blood cells flowing axisymmetrically in a capillary. The elastic constants of the membrane used are $B = 0.0005$ dyn/cm, $D = 10^{-12}$ dyn/cm and $\lambda_i = 0.95$. The unstressed radius of the red cell is 3.91 cm.

have a curvature which is convex upstream indicates that the pressure in the cell lies between the upstream and downstream pressures. Both the front and rear faces are under tension. The role of the bending stress is small except at the sharply curved edges of the cell near the tube wall. These outermost parts of the cell would be bent even more sharply, perhaps even to a cusp if the pressure drop were sufficiently large. For the pressure drops shown in Figs. 8 and 9 the bending of these rear rims is moderate. At higher pressures the computations do not easily converge. It would be suitable to use a membrane without any bending stiffness, but still with constant area in this range. An approximate theory of this type has been suggested by Barnard et al [3].

It may also be noted that the radial movement of any

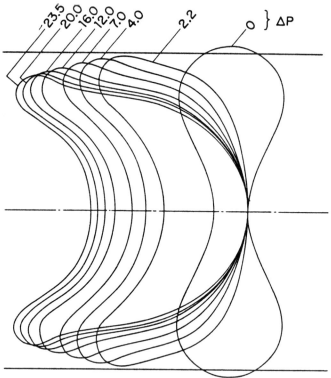

FIG. 9.   Shapes computed for red blood cells
flowing axisymmetrically in a capillary.   The
elastic constants of the membrane used are
B = 0.0005 dyn/cm, D = 10^{-12} dyn/cm and λ_i =
1.05.   The unstressed radius of the red cell
is 3.91 cm.

point on the cell from zero pressure drop to the maximum pressure drop shown in Fig. 8 is not very large
percentagewise.   This indicates that the extensional
strains in the circumferential direction are moderate.
The aximuthal extension ratio is the reciprocal of the
circumferential extension ratio when the area is assumed constant so that it is also near unity.   A certain amount of the stress in the red cell membrane can
be carried out by isotropic tension which is added when
the membrane is assumed to be of constant area.

In performing the computations for the initial diameter ratio, λ_i = 1.05, the cases where the cell nearly touches the wall were computed in a reverse manner;
that is, the shapes at high pressure drops were established first and the pressure drops then gradually reduced until particle membrane approached the tube wall.
When the gap between the cell and the wall became too

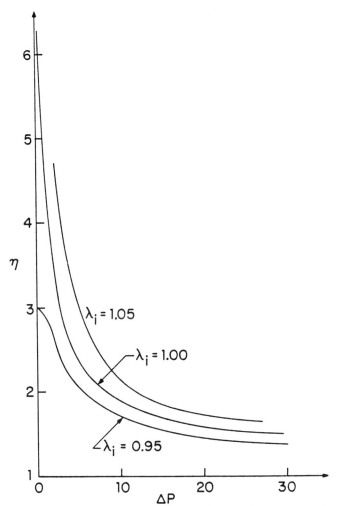

FIG. 10.   Relative apparent viscosity as a function of pressure drop for a line of red blood
cells, as shown in Figs. 1, 8 and 9.

small the computations become unstable.   The results
shown in Fis. 8, 9, 10 are for cases in which a good
convergence and accuracy were obtained.   The characteristic shape in Figs. 8 and 9 showing a flattened
portion of the cell at the rear and more sharply
curved downstream end is due to the typical pressure
distribution outside the cell, similar to that in Fig.
4.   Similar shapes are developed for liquid droplets
as shown by Hyman and Skalak [4].
      The relative apparent viscosity which is found from

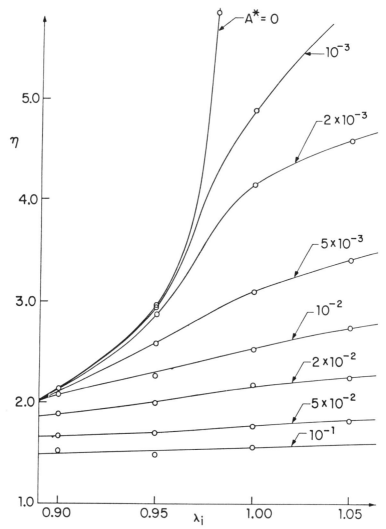

FIG. 11.   Relative apparent viscosity of a line
of red blood cells as shown in Figs. 4, 8 and 9
as a function of the initial diameter ratio and
the velocity parameter A* = μU/B.   The values
for A* = 0 (rigid cells) are derived from Fig. 2.

computations such as shown in Figs. 8 and 9 have a
similar pattern to those of other flexible particles
as shown in Fig. 3.   The relative apparent viscosity
for a hematocrit of 26% is shown in Fig. 11 as a function of the initial diameter ratio λ_i of the tube on
the abscissa and for each curve a dimensionless factor
A* being constant.   The definition of A* is

$$A^* = \frac{\mu U}{B} \tag{16}$$

where B represents the stiffness of the membrane. If b is an assumed thickness of the membrane, the ratio B/b represents an effective shear modulus. The parameter A* may be regarded as a velocity parameter which indicates the relative importance of the shear stresses generated by the flow to the stiffness of the particle. A very stiff particle will behave as a rigid particle and this is the curve labeled A = 0 drawn from the results shown in Fig. 2. The results shown in Fig. 11 are a replotting of the data in Fig. 10 which shows pressure drops on the abscissa for a constant initial diameter ratio λ_i. When the results are plotted as in Fig. 10, it is seen that the apparent viscosity for a given initial diameter ratio will generally decrease as the pressure drop increases. This is because the cells are deformed and thereby pull away from the tube wall. This behavior is similar to that observed in a Couette viscometer in which the apparent viscosity also decreases with increasing shear rate. This is known to be due at least in part to the elastic deformation of the red blood cell (Chien [7]).

The results shown in Fig. 11 are for a hematocrit of about 26% and results for other hematocrits should be computed separately. However, as may be seen in Fig. 2, for particles which occupy most of the tube, the apparent viscosity is nearly linear in H, i.e., $(\eta - 1)$ is proportional to H. This fact may be utilized to predict results up to a hematocrit from zero to about 30% from the results shown in Fig. 11.

The theoretical computational results given in Figs. 10 and 11 are in rough agreement with measurements made on red blood cell suspensions (see Cokelet [9]) in vitro and is vivo (see Lipowsky et al [17]). However, the computed results do not extend to high enough velocities to be realistically compared to in-vivo data which is mostly recorded at higher velocities. Another reason that a close comparison is not possible is that most red cells in actual capillary flows are not axisymmetric as assumed in the computations.

ACKNOWLEDGMENTS

The authors take pleasure in thanking Professor Shu Chien for helpful discussions. The research was made possible by support from National Institutes of Health through research grant HL-16851.

REFERENCES

1. Aroesty, J. and Gross, J.F. (1970): Convection
    and diffusion in the micro-circulation. Micro-
    vasc. Res., 2:247-267.

2. Bagge, U., Skalak, R., Attefors, R. (1977):
    Granulocyte rheology: Experimental studies in
    an invitro micro flow system. Adv. Microcir-
    culation, 1:29-48 (Karger, Basel).

3. Barnard, A.C., Hellums, J.D. and Lopez, L. (1968):
    Basic theory of blood flow in capillaries. Micro-
    vasc. Res., 1:25-34.

4. Bugliarello, O. and Hsiao, C.C. (1967): Numerical
    simulation of three-dimensional flow in the axial
    plasmatic gaps of capillaries. 7th Int. Congress
    Med. Biol. Engng., Stockholm, Sweden.

5. Bungay, P.M. and Brenner, H. (1973): The motion
    of a closely-fitting sphere in a fluid-filled tube.
    Int. J. Multiphase Flow, 1:25-56.

6. Chen, T.C. and Skalak, R. (1970): Spheroidal
    particle flow in a cylindrical tube. Appl. Sci.
    Res., 22:403-441.

7. Chien, S., Usami, S., Jan K.-M. and Skalak, R.
    (1973): Macrorheological and microrheological
    correlation of blood flow in the macrocirculation
    and microcirculation. In: Rheology of Biological
    Systems, edited by H. Gabelnick. M. Litt, 12-48,
    Springfield, Ill.

8. Chien, S., Sung, K.-L.P., Skalak, R., Usami, S.
    and Tozeren, A. (1978): Theoretical and experi-
    mental studies on viscoelastic properties of
    erythrocyte membrane. Biophys. J., 2:463-487.

9. Cokelet, G.R. (1976): Macroscopic rheology and
    tube flow of human blood. Microcirculation,
    edited by J. Grayson and W. Zingg, 1:9-32, Plenum
    Press, New York.

10. Fitz-Gerald, J.M. (1969): Mechanics of red-cell
    motion through very narrow capillaries. Proc.
    Rog. Soc. B 174, 193-214.

11. Goldsmith, H.L. and Mason, S.G. (1971): Theore-
    tical and clinical hemorheology, edited by

H. Hartert and A.L. Copley, 47-59, Springer,
Berlin and New York.

12. Goldsmith, H.L. and Skalak, R. (1975): Hemodynamics. Annual Review of Fluid Mechanics, 7:213-
247.

13. Hochmuth, R.M. and Sutera, S.P. (1970): Spherical caps in low Reynolds number tube flow.
Chem. Eng. Sci., 25:593-604.

14. Hyman, W.A. and Skalak, R. (1972): Non-Newtonian
behavior of a suspension of liquid drops in fluid
flow. A.I.Ch.E. J., 18:149-154.

15. Lew, H.S. and Fung, Y.C. (1969): The motion of
plasma between the red cells in the bolus flow.
Biorheol. 6:109-119.

16. Lighthill, M.J. (1968): Pressure-forcing of
tightly fitting pellets along fluid-filled elastic tubes. J. Fluid Mech., 34:113-143.

17. Lipowsky, H.H., Kovalchech, S., Zweifach, B.W.
(1978): The distribution of blood rheological
parameters in the microvasculature of cat mesentery. Circ. Res., 43:738-749.

18. Skalak, R. (1972): Biomechanics: Its Foundations
and objectives, edited by Y.C. Fung, N. Perrone
and M. Anliber: 457-499, Prentice-Hall,
New Jersey.

19. Skalak, R., Chen, P.H. and Chien, S. (1972):
Effect of hematocrit and rouleaux on apparent
viscosity in capillaries. Biorheol., 9:67-82.

20. Skalak, R., Tözeren, A., Zarda, P.R. and Chien, S.
(1973): Strain energy function of red blood
cell membranes. Biophys. J., 13:245-264.

21. Sutera, S.P. (1977): Red cell motion and deformation in the microcirculation. Cardiovascular
and Pulmonary Dynamics, edited by M.Y. Jaffrin,
71:221-242, INSERM, Paris.

22. Timoshenko, S. and Goodier, J.N. (1951): Theory
of elasticity. McGraw-Hill, New York.

23. Tözeren, H. and Skalak, R. (1978): The steady
flow of closely fitting incompressible elastic

spheres in a tube. J. Fluid Mech., 87:1-16.

24. Tözeren, H. and Skalak, R. (1979): Flow of elastic compressible spheres in tubes. J. Fluid Mech., 95, 4:743-760.

25. Tözeren, H. and Skalak, R. (1979): The flow of closely fitting particles in tapered tubes. Int. J. Multiphase Flow. (In press).

26. Wang, H. and Skalak, R. (1969): Viscous flow in a cylindrical tube containing a line of spherical particles. J. Fluid Mech., 38:75-96.

27. Wohl, P.R. and Rubinow, S.I. (1974): The transverse force on a drop in an unbounded parabolic flow. J. Fluid Mech., 62:185-207.

28. Zarda, P.R., Chien, S. and Skalak, R. (1977): Interaction of a viscous incompressible fluid with an elastic body. Symp. Fluid-Structure Interaction, ASME, New York.

Mathematics of Microcirculation Phenomena,
edited by J. F. Gross and A. Popel.
Raven Press, New York © 1980.

Transluminal Filtration

H. D. Papenfuss and *J. F. Gross

Institute for Thermo and Fluid Dynamics, Ruhr-University Bochum, 4630 Bochum, Federal Republic of Germany, and Department of Chemical Engineering, University of Arizona, Tucson, Arizona 85721

Transluminal filtration is the movement of fluid across the endothelial wall of a capillary from the blood to the extravascular space. The convection of this fluid is responsible for the transport of nutrients and other materials to the organs and individual cells of the body as well as for the removal of metabolic products from the cells. The major driving forces for the fluid flux were first identified by Starling (17) in 1896, and his ideas have dominated the theoretical and experimental work in this area since that time. This review examines and compares the several theoretical approaches that have been used to describe transluminal fluid movement. The review is structured so that a series of models of increasing generality is discussed and compared. A brief description of the experimental approaches used in determining the hydraulic conductivity of the capillary wall is presented. Finally, a summary and forward look discusses the major avenues of experimental and theoretical research in the field of transcapillary fluid exchange to be carried out in the future.

INTRODUCTION

The movement of fluid throughout an organism has always been recognized as a critical element in the maintenance of basic transport processes necessary for life. This fluid movement which is based on the physical principle of convective flow brings water, dissolved low-molecular weight materials, and other substances from the intravascular space through the endothelial wall of the capillaries, through the extravascular tissue to the cells. Two scales of this convective flow may be considered. At the microscopic level, the problem is to describe the motion of the fluid from the lumen of the capillary through the capillary wall into the tissue. At the macroscopic level, one is concerned with the movement of fluid between different organic segments or tissue elements in order to establish an overall fluid movement with-

in an organ. This review will focus on the microscopic phenomena
involved in fluid transport in capillaries and the analytical models which have been formulated in order to explain them. A brief
discussion of the experimental methods to measure the capillary
filtration coefficient will also be presented.

It is clear that the basic description of passive fluid convection in organic systems must follow the appropriate laws of
physics. This was recognized by Ernest Starling (17) who first
proposed a relationship between the transcapillary fluid flux
and the pressure forces. This classical work remains the basis
for the experimental and theoretical work that has been done
since that time. The elaboration of the mathematical statement
of Starling's hypothesis and the important role it plays in the
analytical description of the relationship between the fluid
transport, the hydrostatic and osmotic pressure forces, and the
properties of the capillary walls is the major concern of this
review.

It should be noted from the outset that the analytical models
developed to describe transluminal fluid transport were usually
created in connection with a particular set of experiments and
hence reflected the approach of the experimental technique. The
purpose of these analyses was to create a mathematical framework
within which the data could be most usefully interpreted. More
recently, models have been developed which have attempted to
treat the problem of transluminal filtration more generally and
at least one has led to the formulation of a new experimental
procedure (Blake and Gross (3)). Comparisons between the different analyses will be made and the usefulness of the increasing
generality of the solutions will be evident. It will be seen
that, to the present time, the major approach to the solution of
the governing equations has been the use of the method of asymptotic expansions.

FUNDAMENTAL ASSUMPTIONS

In order to formulate a quantitative description of fluid exchange in the microcirculation, we will focus our attention to a
single capillary as a representation for the entire capillary
network of the tissue. We assume that the capillary has a length L

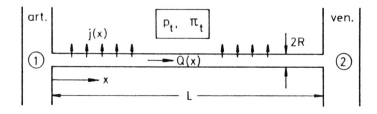

FIG. 1. Geometry of capillary

and a constant radius R; see FIG. 1. The resistance of the capillary wall to transmural fluid flow is embodied in the hydraulic
conductivity K which, in general, depends on the axial position x
along the capillary.

The theory of transcapillary fluid exchange is based on the
hypothesis that the local fluid flux j at an arbitrary axial position x of a capillary is proportional to the local difference
between the transmural hydrostatic and transmural oncotic pressure
drops:

$$j(x) = -K(x) \cdot \{[p(x) - p_t] - [\pi_{pl}(x) - \pi_t]\} \ . \quad (1)$$

Eq. (1) is in the form of Starling's equation where p and π designate the hydrostatic and oncotic pressures, respectively. The
subscript pl stands for plasma and t for the surrounding tissue.
We assume that the capillary is surrounded by a constant milieu;
i.e., we neglect axial variations of the tissue hydrostatic and
oncotic pressures on the scale of the length of a capillary. The
assumption of a constant milieu means also that the values for p_t
and π_t remain unchanged despite fluid transport across the capillary wall. The latter is a reasonable assumption because of the
relatively small filtration or absorption rates which one usually
encounters in most tissues.

It should be noted that Eq.(1) describes only the transmural
flux of fluid, i.e., transmural flux of pure solvent. A similar
equation can be written which accounts for the net transmural
volumetric flux and, hence, includes the flux of proteins across
the capillary wall:

$$j_v(x) = -L_p(x) \cdot \{[p(x) - p_t] - \sigma(x) \cdot [\pi_{pl}(x) - \pi_t]\} \ . \quad (2)$$

In Eq.(2), σ is the so-called reflection coefficient which ex-
presses the transcapillary protein movement and may vary between
O and 1. L_p is a transport coefficient according to the principles of irreversible thermodynamics and should not be con-
fused with the hydraulic conductivity K. The present work is primarily concerned with fluid exchange across semipermeable walls.
In that case, $\sigma = 1$ and the transport coefficients L_p and K are
equal. We consider the hydraulic conductivity K to be a phenomenological coefficient which makes the introduction of fictitious
capillary pores unnecessary.

FORMULATION OF THE PROBLEM OF TRANSCAPILLARY FLUID EXCHANGE

The purpose of investigating the details of transcapillary
fluid movement is to determine the amount of fluid that is filtered or absorbed by the capillary under various physiological
conditions. This means that, in addition to the local value given
in Eq.(1), knowledge of the integral value, i.e., the filtration
rate FR, is of great physiological significance:

$$FR = A \cdot \int_0^1 K(x^*)\{[p(x^*) - p_t] - [\pi_{pl}(x^*) - \pi_t]\}dx^* \quad (3)$$

where $x^* = x/L$ and $A = 2\pi RL$ is the capillary surface area.

It is clear that FR is equal to the difference between the blood volume flows at the arterial and venous ends of the capillary. The dimensionless filtration fraction FF is defined as

$$FF = \frac{FR}{Q_1 \cdot [1 - H_F]} \tag{4}$$

where Q_1 is the volumetric flow rate of blood entering the capillary. H_F is the (feed) hematocrit of the blood entering the capillary. Thus, the denominator of Eq.(4) is equal to the plasma flow rate at the entrance of the capillary.

The major goals of *in vivo* studies of transcapillary fluid exchange are the measurement of FR (or FF) and the determination of $K(x^*)$. However, it must be emphasized that the results of these experimental studies are strictly related to the model that is used to evaluate Eqs.(1), (3) or (4). We will, therefore, present a brief outline of the models for transcapillary fluid exchange which are presently in use. In order to understand the differences between the individual models, it is sufficient to consider the special case of axially-constant hydraulic conductivity.

MODELS FOR TRANSCAPILLARY FLUID EXCHANGE WITH AXIALLY-CONSTANT
HYDRAULIC CONDUCTIVITY

When the hydraulic conductivity K is constant, Eq.(3) reduces to

$$FR = K \cdot A \int_0^1 \{[p(x^*) - p_t] - [\pi_{pl}(x^*) - \pi_t]\}dx^* . \tag{5}$$

We will consider five models based on different assumptions. These will lead to different expressions for FR, and these expressions will vary in complexity depending on the assumptions made.

Model 1:
The assumptions

$$p(x^*) = p_c = const$$

$$\pi_{pl}(x^*) = \pi_{pl} = const$$

lead to

$$FR = K \cdot A \cdot \{[p_c - p_t] - [\pi_{pl} - \pi_t]\} . \tag{6}$$

These assumptions are very restrictive and do not comply with the conservation laws for momentum and mass. The major advantage of the model is its simplicity; its disadvantage is limited accuracy and inability to reflect physiological behaviour. The model has

been used extensively by Wiederhielm (18,19) who modified it
slightly by splitting the capillary into an arterial and a venous
part.

Model 2:
A more realistic approach is to permit the intraluminal hydrostatic pressure to vary linearly along the capillary axis. The
assumptions

$$p(x^*) = p_1 (1 - \omega x^*) \qquad (\omega = const)$$

$$\pi_{pl}(x^*) = \pi_{pl} = const$$

lead to

$$FR = \quad K \cdot A \cdot \{[p_1(1 - \frac{\omega}{2}) - p_t] - [\pi_{pl} - \pi_t]\} \quad . \qquad (7)$$

This equation reflects the classical concept of transcapillary
fluid exchange as expressed in numerous physiological textbooks.
In this case, the capillary filters fluid into the extracapillary
space at the arterial end and reabsorbs it at the venous end.

Model 3:
In this model, the a priori assumption of the behavior of the intraluminal hydrostatic pressure is relaxed and the pressure is
determined from the momentum equation. The plasma oncotic
pressure is assumed to be constant $\pi_{pl}(x^*) = \pi_{pl} = const$. This
leads to an analytical solution:

$$FR = K \cdot A \cdot \{ \frac{\cosh 4\sqrt{\varepsilon} - 1}{2\sqrt{\varepsilon} \cdot \sinh 4\sqrt{\varepsilon}} (\frac{p_1 + p_2}{2} - p_t + \pi_t) - \pi_{pl} \} . \qquad (8)$$

ε is a dimensionless parameter which is defined as

$$\varepsilon = \frac{K \mu}{R} (\frac{L}{R})^2 . \qquad (9)$$

In the following, this parameter will be denoted as fluid-filtration parameter. Its value differs from tissue to tissue but is
usually smaller than 0.01. In Eq.(9), μ is the blood viscosity.
    In the double limit $\varepsilon \to 0$ and $p_E \to p_A$, Eq.(8) becomes identi-
cal to Eq.(6) of Model 1. In the limiting case $\varepsilon \to 0$ and
$p_2 = p_1 (1 - \omega)$, Eq.(8) becomes identical to Eq.(7) of Model 2.
    Model 3 has been used by Apelblat et al. (2) and An and
Salathe (1).

Model 4:
The assumption

$$p(x^*) = p_1 (1 - \omega x^*) \qquad (\omega = const) ,$$

and $\pi_{pl}(x^*)$ resulting from a differential equation that reflects the conservation of the mass of proteins in the capillary lead to

$$FR = K \cdot A \cdot \{p_1(1 - \frac{\omega}{2}) - p_t + \pi_t - \int_0^1 \pi_{pl}(x^*)dx^*\}$$

$$= (1 - H_F) \cdot Q_1 \cdot (1 - c_1/c_2) \ . \tag{10}$$

In this equation, c_1 and c_2 are the plasma protein concentrations at the arterial and venous ends of the capillary, respectively. This model has been used by Deen et al. (5) to study glomerular filtration.

Model 5:
This model does not employ any assumptions regarding $p(x^*)$ and $\pi_{pl}(x^*)$. The hydrostatic pressure $p(x^*)$ is determined by the momentum equation, the oncotic pressure $\pi_{pl}(x^*)$ by the conservation of proteins in the capillary. The latter leads to the following equation for the filtration rate

$$FR = (1 - H_F) \cdot Q_1 \cdot (1 - c_1/c_2) \ . \tag{11}$$

This equation is identical to Eq.(10) except that c_2 is determined in a different fashion. This model leads to a set of coupled nonlinear differential equations which can be solved either numerically or analytically by means of asymptotic perturbation methods. This model has been used by Huss et al. (8), and in a more sophisticated and extended version by Papenfuss and Gross (14) and Papenfuss et al. (15). In contrast to the preceding models, this model retains the major features of the physics in the equations and distinguishes itself through a wider range of application. Therefore, it seems to be appropriate to present the details of this model.

MATHEMATICAL DETAILS OF MODEL 5

By using a mass balance, Eq.(1) can be written as

$$\frac{dQ}{dx^*} = -2\pi R \cdot K \cdot \{[p(x^*) - p_t] - [\pi_{pl}(x^*) - \pi_t]\} \ . \tag{12}$$

It is customary to denote the combination

$$p_e(x^*) = p(x^*) - p_t + \pi_t \tag{13}$$

that appears in Eq.(12) as 'effective pressure'. The local oncotic pressure of the blood can be calculated from the axially varying plasma protein concentration c according to the empirical equation

$$\pi_{pl} = \alpha \cdot c + \beta \cdot c^2 + \delta \cdot c^3 . \tag{14}$$

The coefficients α, β and δ have been reported by Landis and Pappenheimer (10) to be

$$\alpha = 2.1 \frac{mm\ Hg}{g/100\ ml} \ ; \quad \beta = 0.16 \frac{mm\ Hg}{(g/100\ ml)^2} \ ; \quad \delta = 0.009 \frac{mm\ Hg}{(g/100\ ml)^3}$$

The blood volume flow $Q(x^*)$ in Eq.(12) is related to the axial pressure gradient through the generalized Poiseuille equation

$$\frac{dp_e}{dx^*} = - 8 \frac{\mu}{\pi R^4} \ Q(x^*) \tag{15}$$

where μ is the blood viscosity in the capillary. The viscosity of capillary blood is a very complicated function of capillary radius, tubular hematocrit, volume flow, elastic properties of the red cell membrane and plasma protein concentration. Currently, the determination of the blood viscosity in capillaries is the subject of extensive laboratory studies. However, a complete quantitative description of μ as a function of the parameters mentioned above is still lacking, and one is, therefore, forced to assume a reasonable value between 1.4 and 3 cP. It is worth mentioning that Eq.(15) follows from a momentum balance for the flow through a pipe with permeable walls assuming that

$$Re \cdot \frac{R}{L} \ll 1 \quad \text{and} \quad \frac{|j(x^*)|}{Q(x^*)/(R^2\pi)} \ll 1$$

(Re = Reynolds number of axial blood flow).

Conservation of plasma proteins in the blood lumen leads to the following equation for the plasma protein concentration

$$c(x^*) = c_1 \cdot \frac{(1 - H_F)\ Q_1}{Q(x^*) - H_F Q_1} . \tag{16}$$

Eqs.(12) to (16) form a set of coupled nonlinear differential equations which are subject to the boundary conditions

$$\left. \begin{aligned} x^* = 0: \ p_e &= p_1 - p_t + \pi_t \\ Q &= Q_1 \\ c &= c_1 \end{aligned} \right\} \tag{17}$$

Rather than using the volume flow at the capillary entrance one
may prescribe the effective pressure p_{e2} at the venous end of the
capillary, i.e., $x^* = 1$, as a boundary condition. From the numerical solution we obtain the pressure, volume flow and plasma
protein concentration as a function of the axial position x^* .
The totel filtration rate FR follows directly from Eq.(16)

$$FR = Q_1 - Q_2 = (1 - H_F) \cdot Q_1 \cdot (1 - c_1/c_2) \qquad (18)$$

where the subscript 2 stands vor the venous end of the capillary.
    The filtration fraction is

$$FF = \frac{FR}{(1 - H_F)Q_1} = 1 - c_1/c_2 \qquad (19)$$

(FF > O: filtration,   FF < O: absorption).

The filtration rate FR tends to zero when Q_1 approaches zero, i.e.
$p_{e1} \to p_{e2}$. Tn this limit, Eq.(19) is indefinite. Close analysis
shows, however, that the filtration fraction does approach a
finite value as $Q_1 \to O$. Since filtration equilibrium occurs
throughout the entire capillary in the limiting case $Q_1 \to O$,
it follows that

$$p_{e1} = \pi_{pl} = \alpha \, c_2 + \beta \, c_2^{\,2} + \delta \, c_2^{\,3} \, . \qquad (2O)$$

This cubic equation can be solved for c_2 which, subsequently, can
be used in Eq.(19). This particular value of c_2 would be independent of the initial plasma protein concentration c_1 , the hydraulic conductivity, and the hematocrit.
    The equations governing transcapillary fluid exchange can be
nondimensionalized by using the following dimensionless quantities:

$$\left. \begin{array}{ccc}
p_e^{\,*} = \dfrac{p_e}{p_{e1}} & \pi_{pl}^{\,*} = \dfrac{\pi_{pl}}{p_{e1}} & c^* = \dfrac{c}{c_1} \\[3ex]
\alpha^* = \dfrac{\alpha \, c_1}{p_{e1}} & \beta^* = \dfrac{\beta \, c_1^{\,2}}{p_{e1}} & \delta^* = \dfrac{\delta \, c_1^{\,3}}{p_{e1}} \\[3ex]
Q^* = \dfrac{Q \, \mu L}{p_{e1} \, \pi R^4} & FR^* = \dfrac{FR \, \mu L}{p_{e1} \, \pi R^4} & \omega^* = \dfrac{p_{e1} - p_{e2}}{p_{e1}}
\end{array} \right\} \qquad (21)$$

Substitution of Eq.(21) into Eqs.(12-17) yields the following set
of dimensionless equations where, for convenience, the asterisks
are ommitted:

$$\frac{dQ}{dx} = -2 \cdot \frac{K\mu}{R} \left(\frac{L}{R}\right)^2 \cdot [p_e(x) - \pi_{pl}(x)] \qquad (22)$$

$$\frac{dp_e}{dx} = -8 \, Q(x) \qquad (23)$$

$$\pi_{pl}(x) = \alpha \, c(x) + \beta \, c^2(x) + \delta \, c^3(x) \qquad (24)$$

$$c(x) = \frac{Q_1 \, (1 - H_F)}{Q(x) - H_F \cdot Q_1} \qquad (25)$$

The boundary conditions are

$$\begin{array}{lll} x = 0 : & p_e = 1 \, , & c = 1 \\ x = 1 : & p_e = 1 - \omega & . \end{array} \qquad (26)$$

The dimensionless factor

$$\varepsilon = \frac{K\mu}{R} \left(\frac{L}{R}\right)^2 \qquad (27)$$

which appears in Eq.(22) is the fluid-filtration parameter that has already been used in Eq.(8). This parameter plays a key role in transcapillary fluid exchange. Its physical interpretation becomes apparent when Eq.(27) is grouped in the following way

$$\varepsilon = \frac{1}{16} \frac{8\mu L/(\pi R^4)}{(2\pi RLK)^{-1}} \qquad (28)$$

With the exception of the constant factor $1/16$, ε is the ratio between the hydraulic resistance that the capillary wall offers with regard to axial blood flow and the hydraulic resistance of the capillary wall with regard to radial fluid exchange.

If $\varepsilon/\omega \ll 1$, a case that is encountered in the most tissues, a perturbation analysis for $\varepsilon \to 0$ can be done to solve the set of coupled nonlinear differential equations. For this case, we will use the following asymptotic expansions:

$$p_e(x ; \varepsilon) = p_e^{(1)}(x) + \varepsilon \, p_e^{(2)}(x) + \varepsilon^2 p_e^{(3)}(x) + \ldots \qquad (29)$$

$$Q(x ; \varepsilon) = Q^{(1)}(x) + \varepsilon \, Q^{(2)}(x) + \varepsilon^2 Q^{(3)}(x) + \ldots \qquad (30)$$

Introducing these expansions into Eqs.(22-26) and collecting terms of equal power of ε lead to a system of linear differential equations. The analytical solutions for the first three terms of the asymptotic expansions are:

$$p_e^{(1)}(x) = 1 - \omega x \tag{31}$$

$$p_e^{(2)}(x) = -8\left[\frac{\omega}{3}(x^3 - x) - G \cdot (x^2 - x)\right] \tag{32}$$

$$p_e^{(3)}(x) = 256\left\{\frac{G}{2}\left[\frac{x^4}{12} - \frac{x^3}{6} + \frac{x}{12}\right] - \frac{\omega}{6}\left[\frac{x^5}{20} - \frac{x^3}{6} + \frac{7x}{60}\right]\right.$$

$$\left. - \frac{M \cdot G}{6\,\omega}(x^3 - x) + \frac{M}{24}(x^4 - x)\right\} \tag{33}$$

$$Q^{(1)} = \frac{\omega}{8} \tag{34}$$

$$Q^{(2)}(x) = \omega\left(x^2 - \frac{1}{3}\right) - 2G\left(x - \frac{1}{2}\right) \tag{35}$$

$$Q^{(3)}(x) = -32\left\{\frac{G}{2}\left[\frac{x^3}{3} - \frac{x^2}{2} + \frac{1}{12}\right] - \frac{\omega}{6}\left[\frac{x^4}{4} - \frac{x^2}{2} + \frac{7}{60}\right]\right.$$

$$\left. - \frac{M \cdot G}{2\,\omega}\left(x^2 - \frac{1}{3}\right) + \frac{M}{6}\left(x^3 - \frac{1}{4}\right)\right\} . \tag{36}$$

The following abbreviations have been used

$$G = 1 - (\alpha + \beta + \delta) \tag{37}$$

$$M = (\alpha + 2\beta + 3\delta)/(1 - H_F) \tag{38}$$

Using Eqs.(34-36) to determine the filtration rate results in

$$FR = \varepsilon \cdot (2\,G - \omega) + \varepsilon^2 \cdot \left[\frac{4}{3}\omega + \frac{16\,M - 8\,G}{3} - 16\frac{M \cdot G}{\omega}\right] + \dots \tag{39}$$

The leading term of Eq.(39) corresponds to Eq.(7) of Model 2 ; i.e., the error with regard to the filtration rate is of the order of $O(\varepsilon^2)$ for that model. The same is true for Model 4. It is noteworthy that Eqs.(34-36) can be used to determine the axial variation of the plasma protein concentration according to Eq.(25).

APPLICATION OF THE THEORY OF TRANSCAPILLARY FLUID EXCHANGE TO
VARIOUS TISSUES

Rat glomerulus, constant hydraulic conductivity

The capillaries of the renal glomerulus are unique for several
reasons:

1. They are not placed between arterioles and venules but convey
   blood from afferent to efferent arterioles with a concomitant-
   ly small hydrostatic pressure drop.
2. They are not embedded in the interstitium but are bathed by
   the fluid filtrate that is confined in Bowman's capsule.
3. The filtrate is virtually free of plasma proteins in the normal case; i.e., the extravascular oncotic pressure can be set
   equal to zero.
4. The filtration fraction is extremely high.

These physiological properties, however, do not in any way re-
strict the applicability of Model 5. We only replace the subscript t (= tissue) by B (= Bowman's space).

For the numerical computation, the following set of dimensionless parameters were used:

$$\varepsilon = 6.59 \cdot 10^{-3} \quad ; \quad H_F = 0.4 \quad ; \quad Q_1 = 7.66 \cdot 10^{-3}$$

$$\alpha = 0.32053 \quad ; \quad \beta = 0.14164 \quad ; \quad \delta = 0.04621 \quad .$$

These values where calculated from experimental data obtained by
Brenner et al. (4) for surface glomeruli of Wistar rats:
$p_1 = 50$ mm Hg ; $p_B = 12$ mm Hg ; $Q_1 = 2.5$ nl/min ; $K = 3 \cdot 10^{-5}$
cm/(sec $\cdot$ mm Hg). To characterize the capillary geometry and the
intracapillary blood viscosity, the values $R = 4$ μm , $L = 250$ μm
and $\mu = 3$ cP were used.

The axial variations of the intracapillary effective and oncotic pressures as well as of the transmural flux are presented
in FIG. 2. We note that the effective pressure and, therefore,
the hydrostatic pressure decrease virtually linearly along the
capillary axis. The pressure drop along the entire length of the
capillary is about 2 mm Hg ($\omega = 0.051$). In contrast, the oncotic
pressure which is about 50 % of the effective pressure at the
afferent end, increases drastically along the axis due to the
fluid loss and reaches the value of the effective pressure at
about $x/L = 0.75$. Obviously, the assumption of a constant oncotic
pressure would lead to a completely erroneous interpretation of
the transport phenomena in the glomerular capillaries.

The transmural fluid flux which is proportional to the local
difference between the effective and oncotic pressures, decreases
rapidly along the capillary axis. It reaches zero at $x/L \approx 0.75$
(filtration equilibrium) and remains practically zero along the
rest of the capillary. In fact, the theory predicts extremely

small negative values of the flux near the capillary end indicating an insignificantly small amount of reabsorption.

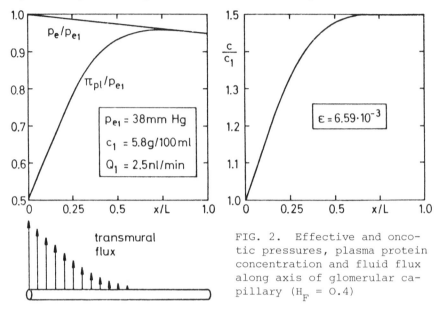

FIG. 2. Effective and oncotic pressures, plasma protein concentration and fluid flux along axis of glomerular capillary (H_F = 0.4)

FIG. 2 shows also the axial variation of the plasma protein concentration due to fluid filtration. The curve corresponds to the axial variation of the oncotic pressure according to the Landis-Pappenheimer equation, Eq.(24). The axial increase of the plasma protein concentration amounts to 50 % which is considerably larger than in other tissues.

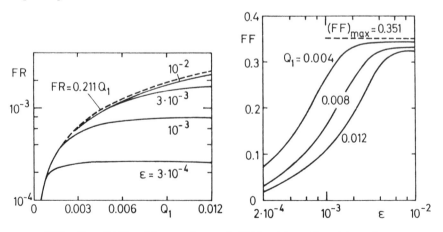

FIG. 3. Filtration rate and filtration fraction for rat glomerular capillary

FIG. 3 shows the influence of the initial blood volume flow Q_1 and the parameter ε on the filtration rate and filtration fraction. All results must unequivocally lie below the dashed curves which are calculated from Eqs.(18-20). For small values of the initial blood flow Q_1, FR is proportional to Q_1 and independent of ε. As Q_1 increases, however, the filtration rate deviates more and more from this linear behavior and tends to a maximum which is a function of the actual value of ε. The appearance of this filtration-rate maximum can be explained with the increasing importance of the oncotic pressure in Starling's equation when the amount of fluid loss due to filtration increases. The curves are rather flat near the filtration-rate maximum; i.e., FR remains almost constant over a wide range of Q_1. In the normal case with $\varepsilon = 6.59 \cdot 10^{-3}$ and $Q_1 = 7.66 \cdot 10^{-3}$, however, changes of Q_1 would be accompanied by almost proportional changes of the filtration rate FR.

FIG. 3 shows that for large values of the filtration parameter ε, the filtration fraction reaches a maximum. The appearance of this maximum could have been predicted from the results for FR which come closer to the dashed line as ε increases. FIG. 3 demonstrates also that the filtration fraction becomes greater with decreasing blood volume flow as has been pointed out earlier.

Rat intestinal muscle, variable hydraulic conductivity

The fluid exchange in the glomerulus described in the previous section is a typical example for extensive filtration. We will now study the opposite case, i.e., that of fluid absorption in the microcirculation of the rat intestinal muscle based on *in-vivo* experiments by Gore et al. (6). These experiments were done with the microocclusion technique at different axial positions along the capillaries which led to a quantitative description of the hydraulic conductivity K as function of the axial coordinate x . The case of axially varying hydraulic conductivity is of great physiological interest since the axial distribution of K can be responsible for the direction of the transmural fluid movement as has been shown by Papenfuss et al. (16).

All the models mentioned before, except Model 1, would be suitable to incorporate axial variations of K . With the modification introduced by Wiederhielm (18,19), even Model 1 can account for axial variations of K by replacing the continuos function K(x) by a step function. In the following, we will present results that have been obtained from Model 5 by using the experimental data of Gore et al. (6) for the variation of the hydraulic conductivity along the axis of capillaries in the rat intestinal muscle.

The values for K at four axial positions averaged over the number of experiments are given in the paper by Gore et al. and are shown in FIG. 4. The solid line in FIG. 4 is a least-squares fit of an exponential function to the experimental data:

$$K/K_{0.5} = 6.686 \, e^{-3.8(1 - x/L)} \tag{40}$$

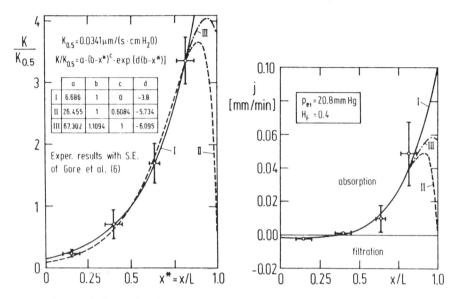

FIG. 4. Axial variation of hydraulic conductivity and transmural
         flux for single capillary of rat intestinal muscle

where $K_{0.5} = 0.0341$ μm/(sec • cm H_2O) is the value at x/L = 0.5 .
Although Eq.(40) fits the experimental data very closely, a problem arises with regard to the venous end of the capillary. For
x/L > 0.82, it is not clear whether the hydraulic conductivity
continues to increase exponentially resulting in K = 0.23 μm/
(sec • cm H_2O) at the venous end, or whether K reaches a maximum
and then approaches zero at x = L. A third case can be postulated
where K reaches a value between 0 and 0.23 μm/(sec • cm H_2O) at
x = L. Because of the design of the experiment used by Gore et al.
(6) it was difficult to occlude the capillaries at the point where
the capillaries enter the venules. Therefore, we examined all
three possible cases and determined the distribution for K from a
nonlinear regression. The resulting equation for K(x) with the
corresponding coefficients are listed in FIG. 4.

     The results of Model 5 for the effective pressure and plasma
oncotic pressure are presented in FIG. 5 as functions of the axial
distance along the capillary. The results for the three cases concerning the distribution of the hydraulic conductivity near the
venous end differ appreciably from each other for the oncotic
pressure but not for the effective pressure. The agreement between
the theoretical results and the experiments of Gore et al. (6)
concerning the effective pressure is shown to be very good.

     The three cases for the hydraulic conductivity function K(x)
which we studied do not cause appreciable differences of the
transmural fluid flux along the first 80 % of the capillary length
as is shown in FIG. 4. At the end of the capillary, however, the
differences between the three cases are large as could be expected

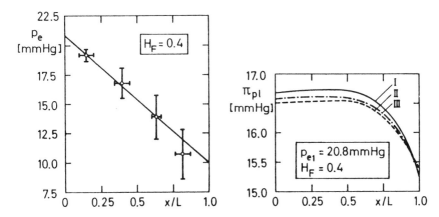

FIG. 5. Axial variation of effective and plasma oncotic pressures in capillary of rat intestinal muscle. Experimental data
with standard errors from Gore et al. (6)

from the uncertainty regarding the axial distribution of the hydraulic conductivity. We notice that for x/L < 0.4 filtration
occurs, but at a low level. The absorption along the last 60 % of
the capillary length clearly dominates the overall rate of fluid
transport. The experimental data with standard errors in that figure are from Gore et al. (6) and were calculated directly from
Starling's equation for four axial positions. The calculations in
that work were based on the experimental results for K, on values
for p_e corrected for the four positions, and on the values for
π_{pl} as determined from samples of the animal's blood. The results
of Model 5, which in contrast is a continuous integration of the
differential equations for axial and radial fluid transport,
agree very well with the experimental data at the four positions.
The differences between the curves for the flux near the venous
end which result from the assumption of three different hydraulic
conductivity distributions have an appreciable effect when the
total filtration rate FR is considered: FR = - 0.053 nl/min with a
range of -0.062 to -0.045 nl/min. Since FR is negative in all
cases, it seems to be certain, despite the lack of experimental
information about the flux near the venous end, that the capillary
bed in the rat intestinal muscle is absorptive.

EXPERIMENTAL DETERMINATION OF THE PERMEABILITY
CHARACTERISTICS OF THE CAPILLARY WALL

It has been mentioned above that a major goal of the experimental research work in fluid exchange across single capillaries
is the determination of the hydraulic conductivity K. Equally important is the determination of the reflection coefficient σ for
plasma proteins. In a recent review, Gore and McDonagh (7) describe and discuss critically the various kinds of microocclusion
techniques which are suitable to determine these crucial para-

meters. All of these techniques are based on the original experiment conducted by Landis (9) which, in contrast to the theory
described above, considers an unsteady phenomenon of transcapillary fluid movement.

Landis-microocclusion (LMO) technique

The Landis experiment which is sketched in FIG. 6 is essentially an occlusion of a single capillary between the arterial
and venous ends with a subsequent analysis of the ensuing migration of the trapped red cells as fluid leaks across the capillary
wall.

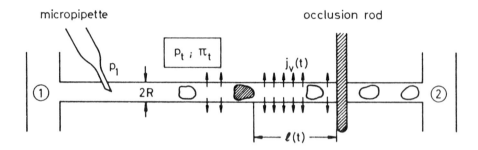

FIG. 6. Microocclusion experiment after Landis (9)

This experiment does not require the assumption that the capillary
wall be semipermeable. In fact, L_p is determined rather than K
with this analysis. The assumptions underlying the LMO-technique
are:

1. No leakage of plasma between the red cell and capillary wall.
2. The volumetric flux j_v is constant along ℓ (see FIG. 6).
3. L_p and σ are independent of the axial position and of the
   hydrostatic pressure.
4. π_{pl} is a function of time only, and independent of the axial
   position.
5. p_t and π_t are constant.

The volumetric flux at the beginning of the occlusion (subscript o) is

$$j_{vo} = -\frac{2R}{4\ell_o} \cdot \left(\frac{d\ell}{dt}\right)_o = -L_p\{[p_1 - p_t] - \sigma[\pi_{plo} - \pi_t]\}$$

(41)

where t is the time. Eq.(41) follows from Eq.(2) and a simple
mass balance. The volumetric flux, j_{vo} , can be determined from
consecutive measurements of the distance ℓ as function of the time

after occlusion; see FIG. 7a. Eq.(41) shows that the derivative of j_{vo} with respect to the occluded pressure p_1 is equal to the coefficient L_p. Therefore, L_p can be determined from consecutive microocclusion experiments with different (= manipulated) values of p_1 ; see FIG. 7b. Although this could be done in a single capillary, Landis (9) examined different capillaries of a tissue that had different occluded pressures p_1 . Thus, Landis avoided the manipulation of the pressure. It is clear that the result from such an experiment represents an average value for the capillaries which have been considered.

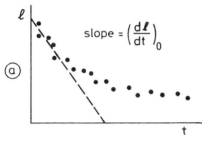

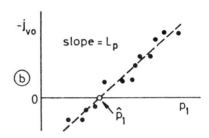

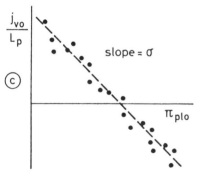

FIG. 7. Data reduction to determine transport coefficients of capillary wall according to the Landis experiment (9)

Although Landis did not determine the reflection coefficient σ, a series of microocclusion experiments with constant pressure p_1 but different values of π_{plo} (injection of an albumin solution into the venous system) would make it possible to calculate σ by taking the derivative of Eq.(41) with respect to π_{plo} ; see FIG.7c.

Michel-microocclusion (MMO) technique

The MMO-technique is based on the same occlusion principle as the LMO-technique except for several differences in the experimental protocol. Michel et al. (12,13) perfuse frog capillaries with a plasma solution of controlled composition by means of a micropipette. Human red cells which are able to pass through the orifice of the perfusion pipette ($\approx$ 10 μm i.d.) serve as markers.

The capillary bed is bathed in a solution in order to control the tissue variables. With this experiment, Michel et al. (12,13) determine both coefficients, L_p and σ , for single capillaries using Eq.(41). However, since frog capillaries are considerably larger in diameter than human red cells, it is very likely that leakage of plasma around the human red cells occurs. Therefore, the results of Michel et al. (12,13) must be considered with some care.

The Lee, Smaje and Zweifach (LSZ) technique

The LSZ-technique (11) is a more sophisticated version of the original LMO-technique with the following modifications:

1. The reflection coefficient σ is assumed to be one; i.e. $L_p = K$.
2. The relative migration of two red cells is observed; see FIG. 8. The volumetric flux j is assumed to be constant only along the distance z(t) between the two red cells under study.

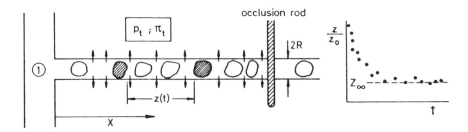

FIG. 8.   Microocclusion experiment after Lee, Smaje and Zweifach (11). Z_∞ = asymptotic distance between erythrocytes, normalized with distance at t = O

Using the definition of the effective pressure, Eq.(13), the volumetric flux can be expressed as

$$j(t) = - \frac{2R}{4z(t)} \cdot \frac{dz}{dt} = - K \cdot [p_{e1} - \pi_{pl}(t)] \ . \tag{42}$$

For $t \rightarrow \infty$, the flux will be zero; i.e.,

$$p_{e1} = \pi_{pl\infty} \ . \tag{43}$$

Lee, Smaje and Zweifach (11) use a quadratic approximation to the cubic Landis-Pappenheimer equation, Eq.(14):

$$\pi_{pl} = \alpha \ c + \beta \ c^2 \tag{44}$$

with α = 2 mm Hg/(g/100 ml) and β = 0.24 mm Hg/(g/100 ml)^2. Since plasma proteins are assumed to be conserved in the lumen, the concentration can be expressed by the distance between the red cells:

$$c(t) = c_o \cdot \frac{1 - H_o}{\frac{z(t)}{z_o} - H_o} \quad , \qquad (45)$$

where the subscript o refers to the time of occlusion, t = 0. H_o is the tubular hematocrit in the capillary segment of length z_o. The occluded effective pressure p_{e1} can now be determined from measurements of H_o, c_o and z_∞/z_o according to Eqs.(43) - (45). See also FIG. 8.

Eq.(42) can be written

$$\frac{1}{Z}\frac{dZ}{dt} = \frac{2K}{R} [p_{e1} - \pi_{pl}(t)] \qquad (46)$$

with Z = z/z_o. The oncotic pressure in Eq.(46) can be replaced by a function of Z according to Eqs.(44) and (45). Evaluation of Eq.(46) at t = 0 would make it possible to calculate K from the equation

$$K = \frac{R}{2} \cdot (\frac{dZ}{dt})_o \cdot \frac{1}{p_{e1} - \pi_{plo}} \quad . \qquad (47)$$

However, Lee, Smaje and Zweifach (11) preferred to solve the differential equation, Eq.(46), using the boundary condition $Z(t \to \infty) = Z_\infty$. This leads to an implicit equation t = f(Z) with H_o, c_o, Z_∞ and K as parameters. A least-squares fit of this equation to the experimental data results in identification of the hydraulic conductivity K. It is noteworthy that the LSZ-method makes it possible to determine K at various positions along the capillary axis as has recently been done by Gore et al. (6) in the rat intestinal muscle.

The Blake and Gross densitometric (BGD) microocclusion technique

It is well-known that changes of the optical density of impermeable intravascular dyes following fluid filtration may be used to determine the hydraulic conductivity K of the capillary wall. Wiederhielm (20,21) was the first to use this densitometric technique to determine the ratio between the hydraulic conductivities of arterial and venous capillaries in the frog mesentery.

In a recent paper, Blake and Gross (3) presented a mathematical description of the pre- and post-occluded flow in single capillaries. That analysis used the method of matched asymptotic expansions where the perturbation parameter

$$\hat{\varepsilon} = \sqrt{\frac{A \cdot K_1 \cdot p_1}{Q_1}} \qquad (48)$$

was based on fluid dynamic characteristics of the pre-occluded flow. The result of the analysis was that changes of the plasma protein concentration c , axial blood velocity v and intravascular pressure p following occlusion are of the order $O(\hat{\mathcal{E}})$, $O(\hat{\mathcal{E}}^3)$ and $O(\hat{\mathcal{E}}^5)$, respectively. This means that the determination of the hydraulic conductivity from densitometric monitoring of the change of the plasma protein concentration will be orders of magnitude more sensitive than observations of the time history of erythrocyte displacements. With the BGD-method the axial distribution of the hydraulic conductivity of a single capillary can be obtained from a single occlusion using the equation

$$\frac{c}{c_1} = 1 + \frac{p_1 - (\alpha c_1 + \beta c_1^2) - p_t(x) + \pi_t(x)}{\alpha c_1 + 2\beta c_1^2} \{1 - $$

$$\exp[- \frac{2K(x)}{R} (\alpha c_1 + 2\beta c_1^2)t]\} \quad . \tag{49}$$

It is noteworthy that the BGD-method even accounts for axial variations of the tissue hydrostatic and oncotic pressures. In fact, all of the assumptions underlying the LMO-technique are relaxed in this method. The only restriction is the assumption of an ideally semipermeable capillary wall. Although the BGD-technique has not yet been applied in experimental studies, it promises to have important advantages over the microocclusion methods presently in use.

SUMMARY AND FORWARD LOOK

The major mathematical formulations for determining the transluminal filtration from a capillary have been presented and discussed. All of them are based on Starling's hypothesis which relates the transluminal filtration flux to the hydrostatic and oncotic pressure driving forces through the hydraulic conductivity coefficient. The restrictions or assumptions upon which each model rests were indicated.

The development of these mathematical models has always been closely aligned with the experimental technique for determining the key parameters in Starling's hypothesis. These experimental methods all derive from the occlusion experiment of Landis (9) and are critically examined in a recent review by Gore and McDonagh (7). It is important, therefore, that the assumptions underlying the experiment be reflected in the analysis used to reduce the data. One key assumption in all of the techniques is that no plasma leaks past the observed erythrocytes in the period subsequent to the occlusion. However, the deformability of the erythrocytes usually permits gaps to appear in the region between the wall of the cell and the endothelial wall. This disturbs the

continuity considerations in the plasma space between the erythrocytes which are a requisite for all of the models for the
post-occlusion flow to the present time. Further theoretical work
to examine the impact of these gaps and plasma leakage on the determination of the hydraulic conductivity coefficient would be a
useful contribution to the theory of transluminal filtration.

The analysis of Blake and Gross (3) demonstrated that the observation of the concentration history of an intraluminal impermeable marker subsequent to an occlusion is a more effective way
to determine the local hydraulic conductivity coefficient than
the classical method of measuring erythrocyte trajectories. This
method has not been demonstrated experimentally. The implications
for ease of measurement and generality in the final results using
such a method are great, and further experimental development of
the technique is an important step in our understanding of transluminal filtration in the microcirculation.

ACKNOWLEDGMENT

We gratefully acknowledge that, while this work was done, one
of us (J.F.G.) was the recipient of an award of the Alexander von
Humboldt-Stiftung, West Germany.

REFERENCES

1. An, K.N., and Salathe, E.P. (1976): The effect of variable
   capillary radius and filtration coefficient on fluid exchange.
   Biorheology 13:367-378.
2. Apelblat, A., Katzir-Katchalsky, A., and Silberberg, A. (1974):
   A mathematical analysis of capillary-tissue fluid exchange.
   Biorheology 11:1-49.
3. Blake, T.R., and Gross, J.F. (1976): Fluid exchange from a
   microoccluded capillary with axial variation of filtration
   parameters. Biorheology 13:357-366.
4. Brenner, B.M., Troy, J.L., Daugharty, T.M., and Deen, W.M.
   (1972): Dynamics of glomerular ultrafiltration in the rat.
   II. Plasma-flow dependence of GFR. Am. J. Physiol. 223:1184-
   1190.
5. Deen, W.M., Robertson, C.R., and Brenner, B.M. (1972): A model
   of glomerular ultrafiltration in the rat. Am. J. Physiol. 223:
   1178-1183.
6. Gore, R.W., Schoknecht, W.E., and Bohlen, H.G. (1976): Filtration coefficients of single capillaries in rat intestinal
   muscle. In: Microcirculation, Vol. 1, edited by J. Grayson and
   W. Zingg, pp. 331-332. Publishing Corp., New York.
7. Gore, R.W., and McDonagh, P.F. (1980): Fluid exchange across
   single capillaries. In: Annual Review of Physiology, edited by
   E. Knobil, (in press). Annual Reviews Inc., Palo Alto, Ca.
8. Huss, R.E., Marsh, D.J., and Kalaba, R.E. (1975): Two models
   of glomerular filtration rate and renal blood flow in the rat.
   Annals of Biomed. Eng. 3:72-99.

9. Landis, E.M. (1927): Micro-injection studies of capillary permeability. II. The relation between capillary pressure and the rate at which fluid passes through the walls of single capillaries. Am. J. Physiol. 82:217-238.
10. Landis, E.M., and Pappenheimer, J.R. (1963): Exchange of substances through the capillary walls. In: Handbook of Physiology, Section 2: Circulation, Vol. 2, Chapter 29. American Physiological Society, Washington, D.C.
11. Lee, J.S., Smaje, L.H., and Zweifach, B.W. (1971): Fluid movement in occluded single capillaries of rabbit omentum. Circ. Res. 28:358-370.
12. Michel, C.C., Baldwin, R., and Levick, J.R. (1969): Cannulation, persusion and pressure measurements in single capillaries in the frog mesentery. In: Techniques Used in the Study of Microcirculation, edited by D.R. Chambers and P.A.G. Munro, pp. 28-32. Plumridge, Linton.
13. Michel, C.C., Mason, J.C., Curry, F.E., Tooke, J.E., and Hunter, P.H. (1974): A development of the Landis technique for measuring the filtration coefficient of individual capillaries in the frog. Quart. J. Exper. Physiol. 59:283-309.
14. Papenfuss, H.D., and Gross, J.F. (1978): Analytical study of the influence of capillary pressure drop and permeability on glomerular ultrafiltration. Microvasc. Res. 16:59-72.
15. Papenfuss, H.D., Gross, J.F., and Thorson, S.T. (1979): An analytical study of ultrafiltration in a hollow fiber artificial kidney. AIChE J. 25:170-179.
16. Papenfuss, H.D., Gore, R.W., and Gross, J.F. (1980): Effect of variable hydraulic conductivity on transcapillary fluid exchange. Application to the microcirculation of rat intestinal muscle. Microvasc. Res. (in press).
17. Starling, E.H. (1896): On the absorption of fluids from the connective tissue spaces. J. Physiol. 19:312-326.
18. Wiederhielm, C.A. (1968): Dynamics of transcapillary fluid exchange. J. Gen. Physiol. 52:29-63.
19. Wiederhielm, C.A. (1979): Dynamics of capillary fluid exchange: A nonlinear computer simulation. Microvasc. Res. 18:48-82.
20. Wiederhielm, C.A. (1966): Transcapillary and interstitial transport phenomena in the mesentery. Fed. Proc. 25:1789-1798.
21. Wiederhielm, C.A. (1967): Analysis of small vessel function. In: Physical Bases of Circulatory Transport: Regulation and Exchange, edited by E.B. Reeve and A.C. Guyton, pp. 313-326. W.B. Saunders Co., Philadelphia.

Mathematics of Microcirculation Phenomena,
edited by J. F. Gross and A. Popel.
Raven Press, New York © 1980.

Mathematical Modeling of Convective and Diffusive Transport in the Microcirculation

*Aleksander S. Popel

*Department of Physiology, College of Medicine, and *Departments of Chemical Engineering and Aerospace and Mechanical Engineering, University of Arizona, Tucson, Arizona 85724*

INTRODUCTION

In order to assess the mechanisms of local regulation of blood flow, it is important to understand the relationship between microvascular network and blood-tissue exchange. It is believed that under normal conditions the capillary blood vessels are the major site of exchange between the blood and the surrounding tissue, although the pre- and post-capillary microcirculation also participate in exchange processes. Mathematical modeling has been proven to be a useful tool in studying various aspects of microcirculatory convective and diffusive transport. The present paper is confined to analyses of particular mathematical models; namely, models of blood flow distribution in branching networks, a model of precapillary oxygen transport in the microcirculation, and models of heterogeneous capillary-tissue oxygen exchange. In addition, a brief review of the experimental findings necessary for understanding the theoretical concepts will be presented.

Many investigators have acknowledged the existence of heterogeneity in the microcirculation, but it was not until recently that careful studies of microvascular morphological and hemodynamic parameters have been conducted. It has been shown that geometrical parameters of microvascular networks such as diameters and lengths of the vessels of a given branching order are heterogeneous, e.g. in skeletal muscle (14, 21, 41). Studies of capillary velocity distribution also reveal wide populations of values (4, 23, 11). In addition to heterogeneity of blood flow, hematocrit in small blood vessels is not uniform from vessel to vessel (22, 50, 51). Possible mechanisms of this phenomenon have been discussed previously (12), and have been studied

in vitro on large-scale models both for the capillary-type (56),
and for the arteriolar-type (3) vessels. Recent studies suggest
that the mean vessel hematocrit (sometimes called "tube hematocrit" or "microvessel hematocrit") falls gradually as blood
approaches the capillaries (33), and the mean capillary hematocrit is within the range 8-20% (24, 31, 33, 50). Several
explanations have been proposed regarding the low capillary
hematocrit phenomenon (24, 33, 46). Since a major fraction of
oxygen carried by the blood is bound to hemoglobin contained inside red blood cells (RBC), the discovered heterogeneity of RBC
volume flux to the capillaries leads to a reconsideration of
Krogh's classical concepts of capillary-tissue oxygen exchange
(25). Studies of oxygen transport in the arteriolar bed have
shown that the oxygen molecules can diffuse through arteriolar
walls and, as a result, oxygen tension (PO_2) falls along the
blood pathway (8, 9, 43). The precapillary oxygen losses have
been shown to be dependent on the blood flow rate (43) and, thus,
on the transit time of blood particles in the arteriolar network.
Therefore, it is clear that PO_2 in the blood particles reaching
the capillaries depends, among other factors, on the particle
pathway in the arteriolar network. In addition to already
mentioned factors affecting the capillary-tissue oxygen exchange
an important factor, at least in skeletal muscle, appears to be
the relationship between the capillary density and the types of
muscle fibers in the same field, e.g., (14).

The complexity of the physiological problems makes mathematical
modeling of these phenomena particularly useful. Review
articles (10, 17, 27, 29) have dealt with some of the theoretical
studies of the described problems. The objective of the present
paper is to disucss recent advances in this area.

MODELING OF FLOW AND PRESSURE DISTRIBUTION IN MICROVASCULAR NETWORKS

The distribution of flow and pressure in microvascular networks is determined by many factors the most important of which
are the topological structure of the network, dimensions of the
blood vessels, and rheological properties of blood. Extensive
theoretical work has been done on the mechanics of blood flow in
single blood vessels, especially the capillaries. The present
paper will focus on the studies of entire networks, which, of
course, include as a necessary element the mechanics of single
vessels. A number of attempts have been made to simulate the
hemodynamics of microcirculatory networks. Schmid-Schonbein and
Devendran (52) used the data of Wiedeman (55) on the number of
vessels, lengths and diameters for the vascular beds in the wings
of unanesthetized bats, to calculate the intravascular pressure
and shear stress distribution in the microvasculature; a simple
model of series-parallel vessel arrangement was considered with
series connection of vessels of different branching order, and

parallel connection of the vessels of the same branching order
(Fig. 1). A characteristic feature of this network is homogeneity of pressure and flow in the vessels of the same branching
order.

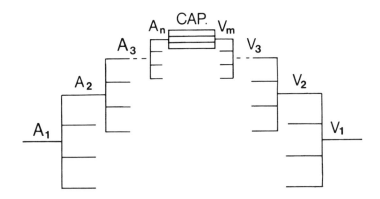

FIG. 1.   Schematic representation of the series-parallel network
model. A = arterioles, CAP. = capillaries, V = venules.

Most subsequent theoretical studies of the microvascular network behavior were concerned with either mesenteric or bat wing
networks. Lee and Nellis (28) considered the vascular pattern of
the mesentery module in the form of a two-dimensional lattice
with five capillary groups and calculated the flow distribution
in this network. A more comprehensive analysis of a single
module of the cat mesentery was done by Lipowsky and Zweifach
(30). Their approach is illustrated in Fig. 2a. A particular
module of the mesentery bounded by paired arterioles and venules
was chosen and the vessels in the model were interconnected in
the same way as in the tissue. For each node in the network the
conservation of mass relationships were written, and Poiseuille's
Law was used to express the volumetric flow rate through each
vascular segment in terms of the pressure difference along the
vessel; blood was considered as a Newtonian fluid. The results
of calculations were compared with experimental measurements of
intravascular pressure (Fig. 2b). The major reason for a discrepancy between the results of computation and in vivo measurements was attributed to the non-Newtonian behavior of the blood.
Other possible factors, such as the hydrodynamic effect of the
bifurcations were also mentioned. Mayrovitz et al. (35) developed a mathematical model of branching networks and applied it to
the bat wing microvascular network. In contrast to the model of
the mesentery, these authors gave a topological description of
the system without attempting to reproduce exactly the interconnections of particular vessels (the topology of the network is

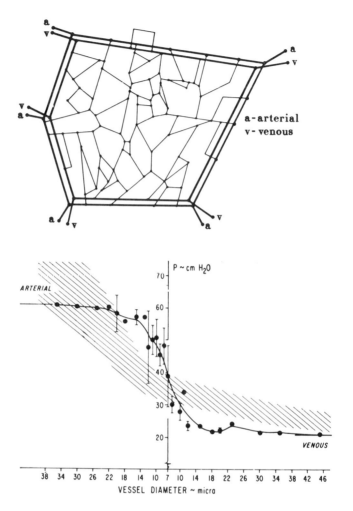

FIG. 2. a. Schematic representation of a typical mesenteric module. Nodes labelled a and v represent boundary nodes for the hydrodynamic computation. b. Distribution of mean intravascular pressure. Computed mean intravascular pressures, averaged at each discrete diameter are represented by the circular symbols bracketed by a band of ± 1σ (where σ equals the standard deviation). Standard deviations less than 1 cm H₂O are not shown. The solid line represents a cubic spline fit of the computed pressures. The cross-hatched area represents the band of intravascular pressures measured in vivo for 150 modules. From (30), reproduced by permission.

illustrated in Fig. 3). Each vessel in the network was represented by a sequence of equal hydrodynamic resistances of the

vascular segments with lateral resistances pertaining to
daughter branches. Recursive relationships for computation of
the entire network hydrodynamic resistance were derived. The
scheme was then used to study the sensitivity of the total hydrodynamic resistance to variations of vessel diameters of different
branching orders (34). The results were presented as the ratio
of resistance to a "control" value. The resistance was most
sensitive to changes in diameter of the large vessels with control diameters of about 100μ, and showed a decrease in the degree
of sensitivity as the branching order increased. The total
resistance was practically insensitive to dilation of terminal
arterioles (about 5μ in diameter), but was sensitive to con-
striction of these vessels, although to a lesser degree than for
the larger vessels. Mayrovitz et al. (36) also applied their
model to calculate the distribution of the mean flow and pressure
in the network; the results on the pressure distribution were
shown to be in agreement with experimental data.

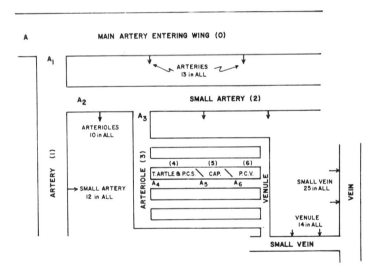

FIG. 3. Topological model of the bat wing microcirculatory network. One pathway from main artery to small vein is shown in
detail, and the remainder of the branches and vascular pathways
are shown in straight arrows. Numbers in parentheses designate
the branching order. ARTLE = terminal arteriole, P.C.S. =
precapillary sphincter, CAP. = capillary, P.C.V. = postcapillary
venule. From (34), reproduced by permission.

Inherent to the branching geometry of the network is heterogeneity of hemodynamic parameters, such as the pressure and
flow, in the vessels of the same branching order. Popel (47)

utilized the morphological data for the bat wing microvasculature
to calculate the flow and pressure in all segments of the network, and presented the results in the form of the frequency
distributions of hemodynamic parameters in vessels of different
branching orders.   The first step in developing a model of
microcirculatory flow is to define the topology of the vascular
network, i.e. to describe the interconnections of vessels of
different branching orders.   It should be noted that this is not
by all means a trivial task because any real structure contains
"random" elements that are not easy to classify.   Two different
approaches to the problem can be employed: the approach of
Lipowsky and Zweifach (30) which due to computational difficulties is limited to networks with a few hundred vessels, and the
approach of Mayrovitz et al. (35) which considers more "regular"
structures.   It appears that the first approach may be most
effective when applied to tissues with "irregular" morphological
structure such as mesentery, whereas the second one may be more
appropriate when applied to tissues with a structure such as in
skeletal muscle.   Illustrated below is a scheme of calculations
for the case of "regular" geometry of the network.   Neglecting
random factors in topology of the network, we can present the
diverging structure of the arteriolar part of the network as
shown in Fig. *4*.

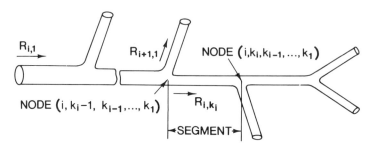

FIG. *4*.   Structure of the *i*th order vessel with illustration of
the notation.

It is assumed that all arteriolar vessels of an *i*th branching
order are geometrically identical (therefore, neither topological nor geometrical randomness are taken into account).   Each
vessel of the *i*th branching order contains M_i segments.
Segments of the same vessel are not necessarily identical and
following each bifurcation the diameter of the vessel may be
reduced (tapering of the vessel).   Each node in the network can
be identified by a sequence $(i, k_i, k_{i-1}, \ldots, k_1)$, where the index
i refers to the branching order of the vessel, k_i is the number
of nodes preceding a given node in the given vessel, and the
sequence $(i-1, k_{i-1}, k_{i-2}, \ldots, k_1)$ characterizes the node from which
the vessel originates.   The hydrodynamic pressure at the node

$(i,k_i,k_{i-1},\ldots,k_1)$ is denoted as $p_{i,k_i,k_{i-1},\ldots,k_1}$, and the volumetric flow rate in the segment preceding this node is denoted as $Q_{i,k_i,k_{i-1},\ldots,k_1}$. The conservation of mass relationships can now be written for each node in the form

$$Q_{i,k_i,k_{i-1},\ldots,k_1} = Q_{i,k_i+1,k_{i-1},\ldots,k_1} + Q_{i+1,1,k_i,\ldots,k_1} \qquad (1)$$

(except for the terminal nodes where the form of the relationship is different), and the momentum equations - for each segment. At this point, the rheological properties of blood come into play. It is known that the apparent viscosity of blood for the flow in cylindrical tubes depends upon such parameters as the "feed" hematocrit, diameter of the tube and the shear rate; a comprehensive analysis of in vitro hemorheology can be found in review papers by Schmid-Schonbein (53) and Cokelet (5). Recently, Lipowsky et al. (32, 33) obtained the data on apparent viscosity of blood in vivo taking measurements of pressure drop in single vessels in the cat mesentery. The difficulty in applying the information on blood viscosity obtained in vivo or in vitro, to the branching network model lies in yet unknown relationships between the values of hematocrit in the segments adjacent to each network node. A recent study (51) predicts the hematocrit values in segments downstream from a bifurcation if the red blood cell distribution in the cross-section of the parent vessel is known. This notion, however, is not sufficient for determination of hematocrit in consecutive segments of the network. Thus, at the present time, there is not enough data on the mechanics of red blood cell separation at bifurcations and on concomitant changes in viscosity, to develop a comprehensive theory of blood flow in branching networks. We must resort to a simple rheological model assuming either constant viscosity of blood throughout the arteriolar network (c.f. (32)), or adopting certain relationships between the apparent viscosity and the vessel diameter and systemic hematocrit (5, 33). In view of the observation of Palmer and Betts (42) that the entry region for hematocrit distribution is at least one hundred times the vessel diameter, the apparent viscosity may also be a function of the length of the vascular segment. It appears that under normal flow conditions the shear rates in the arteriolar network are sufficiently high so that the apparent viscosity can be assumed to be independent of the shear rate. With the adopted assumptions regarding the apparent viscosity, the hydrodynamic resistance of a segment is only dependent on the geometric dimensions of the segment and on the systemic hematocrit; if it is further assumed that the segments of the same "order" have identical geometric dimensions despite possible differences in the intravascular pressure then the momentum equation for each segment can be written in the form

$$p_{i,k_i-1,k_{i-1},\ldots,k_1} - p_{i,k_i,k_{i-1},\ldots,k_1} = \quad (2)$$

$$= \zeta_{i,k_i} Q_{i,k_i,k_{i-1},\ldots,k_1}.$$

where $\zeta_{i,j}$ is the hydrodynamic resistance of the segment. The arterial pressure at the inlet of the network, p_a, and the pressure at the outlet of the network, p_v, are specified. The problem, therefore, is in using the linear set of governing equations of the type *(1)* and *(2)* to determine the distribution of pressures in all nodes and the volumetric flow rates in all segments of the network. Real microvascular networks contain thousands of vessels so even the solution of the set of linear algebraic equations becomes a cumbersome problem. A method of auxiliary input hydrodynamic resistances proposed by Mayrovitz et al. (35) leads to a solution of the problem. For the sake of simplicity, in the present analysis the converging venular network is not considered; instead, the capillaries and venules are "lumped" into a terminal resistance $R_{n,1}$ which has to be specified. In this case, the upstream input resistances can be calculated using recursive relationships (see Fig. *4*)

$$R_{i,k_i} = \zeta_{i,k_i} + \frac{R_{i,k_i+1} R_{i+1,1}}{R_{i,k_i+1} + R_{i+1,1}} \quad (3)$$

with appropriate modifications for terminal segments. Thus, the input resistances are calculated step-by-step starting from downstream and finishing with the resistance of the entire network, $R_{1,1}$. The values of flow and pressure can then be calculated in the reverse order, from upstream to downstream. Namely, the first steps are

$$Q_{1,1} = \frac{p_a - p_v}{R_{1,1}}, \quad p_{1,1} = p_a - \zeta_{1,1} Q_{1,1}. \quad (4)$$

Generally, if the flow $Q_{i,k_i-1,k_{i-1},\ldots,k_1}$ and the pressure $p_{i,k_i-1,k_{i-1},\ldots,k_1}$ have already been determined, the flow and pressure further downstream can be found from the following relationships

$$Q_{i,k_i,k_{i-1},\ldots,k_1} = \frac{R_{i+1,1}}{R_{i,k_i} + R_{i+1,1}} Q_{i,k_i-1,k_{i-1},\ldots,k_1}, \quad (5)$$

$$Q_{i+1,1,k_i,\ldots,k_1} = \frac{R_{i,k_i}}{R_{i,k_i} + R_{i+1,1}} Q_{i,k_i,k_{i-1},\ldots,k_1} , \qquad (6)$$

$$P_{i,k_i,k_{i-1},\ldots,k_1} = P_{i,k_i-1,k_{i-1},\ldots,k_1} - $$

$$- \zeta_{i,k_i} Q_{i,k_i,k_{i-1},\ldots,k_1} . \qquad (7)$$

Again, for the terminal segments these relationships require certain modifications.

The above method is employed to calculate the distribution of flow and pressure in the arteriolar network of the bat wing utilizing morphological data (55, 35). Other parameters used in simulation are: viscosity μ = 3cP, terminal resistance $R_{5,1}$ = 3 x 10^{12} dynes/cm^5 sec, arterial pressure p_a = 90 mm Hg, venous pressure p_v = 10 mm Hg. Fig. 5 presents a histogram of the calculated volumetric blood flow rate in the fifth order arterioles (7800 fifth order vessels were considered). The heterogeneity of arteriolar volume flow is born by the branching structure of the network which contains pathways of different lengths. A longer pathway generates a larger precapillary pressure drop, and, hence, a smaller arteriolar flow. The branching structure of the network is only one of the many factors responsible for heterogeneity of the flow in the living tissue. Another important factor is the heterogeneity within any given branching order of geometrical parameters of the vessels. Obviously, the large differences in capillary perfusion mean significant inhomogeneity in oxygen delivery to the tissue; the problem of mathematical modeling of capillary-tissue oxygen exchange under these conditions will be considered in the last section of this paper.

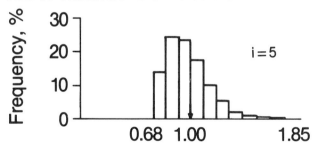

FIG. 5. Frequency distribution of the dimensionless volumetric flow rate at the entrance to the arterioles of the fifth branching order, $Q_{5,1,k_4,\ldots,k_1}/Q_{5,1}$, where $Q_{5,1}$ is the mean value of the flow in the population of all fifth order arterioles.

Fig. *6* presents the frequency distribution of the calculated transit times for the arteriolar network. The transit time is defined here as the time that it takes for an average liquid particle to traverse the distance between the entrance of the first order vessel and the entrance of a fifth order vessel. The width of the distribution reflects the differences in transit times along different pathways in the arteriolar network. It should be noted that the calculated transit times are very long as a consequence of the low flow in this network (36).

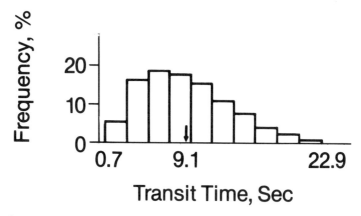

FIG. *6*. Frequency distribution of the transit times in the arteriolar network confined between the network entrance and the entrances of the arterioles of the fifth branching order. The arrow indicates the mean transit time.

The demonstrated approach to the modeling of flow phenomena in branching networks yields the results that are a step forward as compared to the predictions of a series-parallel network model. It is clear, however, that for an adequate description of the system some additional factors have to be taken into account. There are principal mathematical difficulties that must be resolved for further development of the model. The analyses discussed were limited to considerations of linear relationships between the intravascular pressure and blood flow. It can be expected, however, that because the vascular walls are compliant, the vascular diameter and, hence, the hydrodynamic resistance of a vascular segment are dependent on the intravascular pressure. A network model accounting for such an effect would be described by a nonlinear set of equations. In addition, taking into account non-Newtonian properties of blood which may be particularly important for the venular part of the network, as well as separation of red blood cells at bifurcations would result in a nonlinear network model.

Some aspects of time-dependent flow phenomena in microvascular networks were considered by Gross et al. (15), and Mayrovitz et al. (37); compliance of the vascular walls was taken into account. The hydrodynamic effects of the pressure pulsations introduced by the heart and of self-sustained vasomotions were discussed.[a]

PRECAPILLARY OXYGEN LOSSES IN MICROCIRCULATION

The significance of precapillary oxygen transport in the microcirculation was first demonstrated by Duling and Berne (8) who discovered longitudinal gradients in periarteriolar oxygen tension in the hamster cheek pouch. Subsequently, Duling and Pittman (9) have shown that the percentage of oxyhemoglobin in blood decreases along the arteriolar network. It has been suggested (9) that precapillary oxygen transport phenomena may play a role in the local regulation of blood flow. Therefore, it is important to study the effect of such factors as the blood flow rate, vessel geometry, systemic PO_2, blood hematocrit, and oxygen saturation of hemoglobin on the precapillary oxygen losses. We have developed a mathematical model of oxygen exchange between an arteriolar network and the surrounding perfused tissue and made an attempt to simulate the precapillary transport in the hamster cheek pouch (48). Such a model can also assist in understanding the transport phenomena in the deep tissue layers; it appears that the existing experimental techniques are not appropriate for such measurements. In the present section we outline the development of the theory, and show some of the theoretical predictions pertaining to the hamster cheek pouch microcirculation.

First, the problem of oxygen exchange between a single arteriolar vessel and the surrounding tissue is considered, and then the results are applied to a simple series-parallel vascular network. Consider a vessel immersed in an unbounded perfused tissue and formulate equations governing the transfer of oxygen between the lumen of the vessel and the region occupied by the extravascular structure. Theoretical and experimental evidence suggests that the O_2 distribution is nearly uniform in a cross-section of arteriolar vessels due to significant "mixing" in shear flow. An analysis of the mechanisms of oxygen transfer in the axial direction shows that, under normal flow conditions, axial diffusion in blood is negligible in comparison with convection. Thus, the equation of steady-state intraluminal convective transport of oxygen can be written in the form

---

[a] During preparation of the paper two manuscripts appeared in press that are pertinent to the problems discussed in this section. These are:

Levitt, D. G., Sircar, B., Lifson, N., and Lender, E. J. (1979): Model for mucosal circulation of rabbit small intestine. Am. J. Physiol., 237:E373–E382.

Shea, S. M. (1979): Glomerular hemodynamics and vascular structure. The pattern and dimensions of a single rat glomerular capillary network reconstructed from ultrathin sections. Microvasc. Res., 18:129–143.

$$Q\alpha_b \frac{\partial}{\partial x} \{P + N\alpha_b^{-1}\Psi(P)\} = -2\pi R_i J, \qquad (8)$$

where Q is the volumetric flow rate, α_b is the solubility coefficient of oxygen in the blood, x is the coordinate along the
vessel axis, P is the luminal PO_2, N is the O_2-binding capacity
of blood, Ψ is the oxygen saturation fraction of hemoglobin, R_i
is the internal radius of the vessel, and J is the local oxygen
flux at the blood-wall interface. The oxygen distribution in the
vascular wall is described by the equation

$$D_w \alpha_w \frac{1}{r} \frac{\partial}{\partial r} (r \frac{\partial P_w}{\partial r}) - M_w = 0, \qquad (9)$$

where D_w is the oxygen diffusivity in the wall, α_w is the oxygen
solubility coefficient, r is the radial coordinate, P_w is the
oxygen tension in the wall, and M_w is the oxygen consumption
rate. Diffusion in the axial direction within the vascular wall
has been neglected because its effect is small in comparison with
the radial diffusion. The problem of mathematical derivation of
an oxygen transport equation in the vicinity of the arteriolar
vessel taking into account the specific local geometry of the
capillary structure and of the capillary flow is a formidable
task. In fact, even the necessary morphological information is
not presently available. Therefore, we have to resort to less
detailed "phenomenological" modeling of oxygen exchange in the
extra-arteriolar region. The model does not account for hetero-
geneities of PO_2 on the scale of single capillaries and cells
but rather is concerned with "large-scale" diffusional processes
in the vicinity of such sources or sinks of oxygen as arterioles
or venules. Far from such sources or sinks, the model yields an
average PO_2 level, P_∞, which is solely determined by the
capillary-tissue exchange. The simplified linear "diffusion"
equation has the form (in the case of cylindrical symmetry and
with the axial diffusion neglected)

$$\frac{1}{r} \frac{\partial}{\partial r} (r \frac{\partial P_t}{\partial r}) - \ell_t^{-2} (P_t - P_\infty) = 0 \qquad (10)$$

in which P_t is the tissue PO_2, and ℓ_t is a phenominological
parameter with the meaning of a penetration depth.

Equations *(8)* – *(10)* can be solved with appropriate boundary
conditions that require continuity of PO_2 and of the oxygen flux
at the blood-vascular wall and wall-tissue interfaces. In addition, oxygen tension at the entrance of the vessel has to be
specified. The question now arises whether or not the solution
obtained for a single arteriolar vessel is applicable to a vessel which is a part of a network. It can be shown that diffusional interaction between the arteriolar vessels is unimportant if
the average distances between the vessels are several times
larger than the penetration depth ℓ_t. In this case, the obtained

mathematical solution can be used in calculations of PO_2 distribution along the arteriolar network provided that certain relationships between effluent and inlet oxygen tensions in successive branching orders are specified. In principle, the analysis of PO_2 distribution can be combined with one of the branching network models described in the preceding paragraph. In the present example a scheme is adopted that simplifies the computations significantly; namely, a simple series-parallel arrangement of the vessels such that the vessels of successive branching orders are arranged in series, and vessels of the same order are arranged in parallel. Thus, if x_i is the axial coordinate along the vessel of the ith branching order such that $x_i=0$ corresponds to the vessel inlet, then

$$P_i(x_i=L_i) = P_{i+1} (x_{i+1}=0),\qquad(11)$$

where L_i is an effective length of the vessel. Starting with a given luminal PO_2 at the end of the "zeroth" branching order, P_a, and integrating equations sequentially for P_1, P_2, ... using the matching condition *(11)*, one can determine the PO_2 distribution throughout the network.

Some theoretical predictions based on morphological parameters and the values of the blood flow rate pertaining to the hamster cheek pouch microcirculation are given below. It should be realized, however, that the model is only a first approximation to the complex phenomena of the precapillary oxygen transport and many assumptions made for the sake of simplicity may and should be relaxed. In particular, the model does not account for oxygen exchange between the tissue and a superfusion solution which may be of importance under experimental conditions (8, 9). Also, not all parameters used in the model have been measured in the hamster cheek pouch preparation; some of them are taken from observations in other tissues, and some of them, like the penetration depth ℓ_t, remain somewhat uncertain. Therefore, the theoretical predictions are meant to give not a quantitative but rather a qualitative description of the phenomena.

Distributions of the luminal PO_2 and the saturation fraction of hemoglobin Ψ in four successive branching orders of the arteriolar network are plotted in Fig. *7* for various values of the penetration depth.

Fig. *8* shows the variation of intraluminal PO_2 in vessels of different branching orders for various values of the systemic oxygen tension P_a. For high values of P_a ($P_a > 120$ mm Hg) the model predicts that the oxygen tension in small arterioles becomes insensitive to variation of P_a; PO_2 in small arterioles is maintained at the level around 40 mm Hg. On the contrary, for low values of P_a ($P_a < 40$ mm Hg) the precapillary longitudinal gradients practically vanish, i.e. the oxygen tension in small arterioles equals the inlet network oxygen tension P_a.

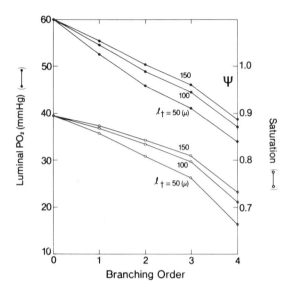

FIG. 7. Distribution of the luminal PO_2 (closed circles) and the saturation fraction of hemoglobin Ψ (open circles) in the arteriolar network for three different values of the penetration depth. From (48), reproduced by permission.

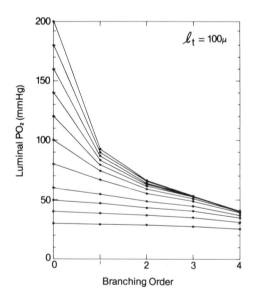

FIG. 8. Distribution of the luminal PO_2 for different values of the inlet network PO_2. From (48), reproduced by permission.

Important features which have not been taken into consideration in the present development include the diffusional interaction between the paired arterioles and venules (44), the
correlation between the transmural diffusion and the "background"
oxygen tension P_∞, and the effect of the tissue surface on transport processes. It can also be expected that for high values of
the inlet network PO_2 the axial diffusion in the blood and in the
tissue may become important; in this case additional terms in the
diffusion equations ought to be considered. A more accurate
analysis should also consider the description of transport from
the terminal arterioles (comparable with capillaries in diameter)
for which the phenomenological approach may not be appropriate,
and probably, should account for unidirectional capillary flow or
flow in a preferential direction in the vicinity of arterioles
of different order.

MATHEMATICAL MODELS OF STEADY-STATE CAPILLARY-TISSUE OXYGEN EXCHANGE

The transport of oxygen between capillary blood vessels and
surrounding tissue structures has been studied extensively both
theoretically and experimentally. Recent review articles by
Leonard and Jorgensen (29), Grunewald and Sowa (17) and Fletcher
(10) contain numerous references of theoretical studies in this
area.
The first simple mathematical model of oxygen exchange was
proposed by Krogh (25). The model is based on a concept that
oxygen from a capillary diffuses only into a tissue cylinder
concentric with the capillary so that the oxygen flux at the
external surface of the cylinder vanishes. Krogh's model, due to
its relative simplicity, has been widely used in physiological
studies to assess the oxygen supply conditions. A large body of
literature is devoted to analyses of oxygen diffusion within the
framework of the Krogh tissue cylinder concept, using both
numerical and analytical techniques (29, 17, 10).
Krogh's geometrical concept of identical parallel capillaries
surrounded by identical tissue cylinders seems to be most appropriate for the skeletal muscle microcirculation with its
"regular" structure. However, recent studies have demonstrated
that the predictions of the model do not agree with experimental
data (19, 20). The cause of this inconsistency may be the fundamental assumption inherent to the Krogh model that the adjacent
capillaries do not interact with each other. This assumption
does not appear justified in view of the recent observations of
morphology and hemodynamics of the microcirculation. Indeed,
morphological studies of capillary networks in longitudinal
(parallel to the capillary axes) and transverse (perpendicular to
capillary axes) sections indicate significant heterogeneity in
the capillary structures as well as the correlation of the
capillary geometry with the location of muscle fibers of different types (14, 41, 21). Significant heterogeneity exists in

tissue perfusion at the capillary level which manifests itself
in heterogeneity of capillary flow (4, 23, 11), and capillary
hematocrit (22, 50, 51). Additionally, the precapillary oxygen
losses discussed in the preceding paragraph may result in heterogeneity in the degree of oxygenation of the blood entering the
capillaries. Therefore, it is clear that the Krogh cylinder
model is a first approximation to the complex phenomena, and the
description of more realistic situations requires models with
diffusional interaction between the capillaries.

Mathematical models different from the Krogh cylinder model
have also been considered. The first steps taking into account
the capillary interaction were made by Diemer (7), Bailey (2),
and Reneau and Knisely (49) who considered different models of
mass transfer under countercurrent flow conditions. It was suggested that countercurrent flow provides a more homogeneous
supply to the tissue than concurrent flow does. Metzger (38, 39)
has considered oxygen diffusion from two- and three-dimensional
capillary structures in the form of square or cubic lattices, the
latter intended to simulate capillary structure in the brain.
The geometry of the cubic lattice is illustrated in Fig. 9; due
to symmetry of the capillary structure, only a tetrahedron outlined in the figure can be examined for a complete description of
the network. Metzger employed numerical techniques to solve a
set of differential equations that allowed him to consider nonlinear relationships for the oxygen dissociation curve and for
the oxygen consumption rate in the tissue. An important feature
of this model is a possibility to study the impact of inhomogeneous capillary perfusion on the distribution of oxygen in the
tissue. Recently, Metzger applied the two-dimensional square
lattice model to study the effect of spatially inhomogeneous
oxygen consumption on oxygen distribution in the tissue (40).

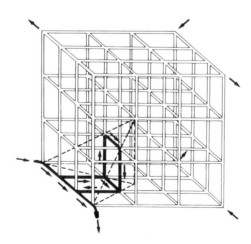

FIG. 9. Capillary-tissue model with outlined tetrahedron. From
(39), reproduced by permission.

Grunewald's model (16; see Fig. *10*a) consists of four parallel capillaries situated along the side of a rectangular parallel-epiped; the inlets and outlets of different capillaries may be situated in different planes that allows for consideration of countercurrent and, generally, asymmetric flow conditions. Grunewald and Sowa (17) describe in detail results of their numerical simulation of oxygen distribution in both resting and exercised skeletal muscle based on Grunewald's model. An example of calculations is reproduced in Fig. *10*b together with experimental data of Kunze (26). Although the authors have been able to closely fit the experimental histograms of PO_2 distribution in the tissue, the choice of parameters made to obtain the fit was only one of the many possibilities. Therefore, the results leave some freedom for interpretation. The model has also been applied to the problem of oxygen transport in the heart (18) and tumors (54).

a.   b.

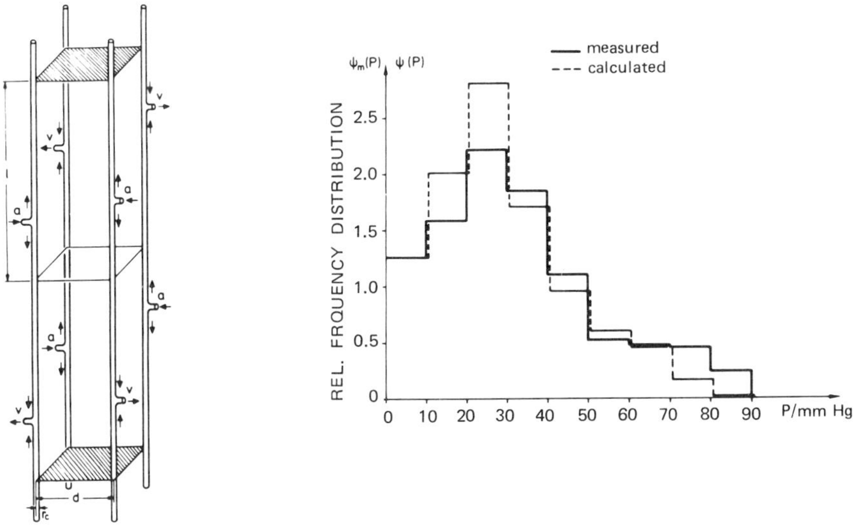

FIG. *10*,a. Basic microcirculatory unit that consists of tissue fragment and four parallel-running capillaries. b. PO_2 distribution $\Psi_m(P)$ measured by Kunze (26), and PO_2 distribution $\Psi(P)$ calculated as a combination of PO_2 distributions for the microcirculatory units with different structure, including the ones with countercurrent flow. From (17), reproduced by permission.

Recently, Popel (45) has made an attempt to extend the model of Grunewald to the case of an arbitrary number of parallel capillaries situated within a parallelepiped; to illustrate the geometry, a cross-section perpendicular to the capillary axes is shown in Fig. *11*.

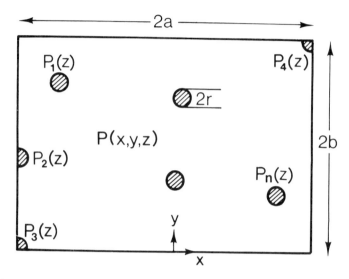

FIG. *11*.   Geometrical distribution of capillaries in the representative rectangle.

The oxygen flux at the boundaries of the parallelepiped is assumed to be zero which implies a certain symmetry of the capillary structure with respect to the boundaries. The intracapillary PO_2 is assumed to be dependent on the axial coordinate z only; calculations done by Aroesty and Gross (1) corroborate this assumption, as well as recent findings of Gaehtgens et al. (13) who observed "tanktreading" of erythrocytes in glass capillary tubes that should lead to additional intraluminal mixing. The axial diffusion in the capillary under normal conditions is negligible compared to convection. Thus, the equations of convective transport of oxygen along the capillaries can be written in the form

$$Q_i \alpha_b \frac{d}{dz} \{P_i + N_i \alpha_b^{-1} \Psi(P_i)\} = - J_i; \quad i = 1, 2, \ldots, n, \quad (12)$$

where Q_i is the volumetric blood flow rate, P_i is the oxygen tension in the ith capillary, and J_i is the capillary-tissue diffusion flux per unit length of the capillary. Other notation has been introduced in the preceding section. If the ratio of a characteristic intercapillary distance to the capillary length is sufficiently small then the axial diffusion in the tissue can be neglected in comparison with diffusion in the x-y plane, (17). In this case the diffusion in the tissue region is governed by the equation

$$D\alpha \left(\frac{\partial^2 P}{\partial x^2} + \frac{\partial^2 P}{\partial y^2}\right) - M = 0, \tag{13}$$

where D is the oxygen diffusion coefficient in the tissue, α is the solubility coefficient of oxygen in the tissue, P is the oxygen tension, and M is the oxygen consumption rate. In addition to the no-flux boundary condition at the boundaries of the rectangle shown in Fig. 11, certain conditions have to be satisfied at the boundary of each capillary Γ_i, namely, the oxygen tension and the oxygen diffusion flux have to be continuous:

$$P = P_i \text{ and } J_i = D\alpha \int \frac{\partial P}{\partial n} \, d\Gamma_i. \tag{14}$$

Equations (12) and (13), with boundary conditions (14) and additional boundary conditions specifying the inlet capillary oxygen tensions, can be solved numerically for a nonlinear dependence of the oxygen consumption rate M on the local tissue PO_2. However, in order to obtain an analytical solution to the problem we limit the consideration to a constant oxygen consumption rate. In this case equations (12) and (13), with boundary conditions (14), can be satisfied approximately making use of the small ratio of the capillary radii to intercapillary distances. The solution can be presented in the form

$$P(x,y,z) = \frac{Mx^2}{2D\alpha} + \frac{Ma^2}{2\pi D\alpha K} I(\xi,\eta) -$$

$$- \frac{1}{4\pi D\alpha} \sum_{i=1}^{n} J_i^* \ln\left[(\xi-\xi_i)^2 + (\eta-\eta_i)^2\right]\left[(\xi-\xi_i)^2 + (\eta + \eta_i)^2\right] + P_o(z), \tag{15}$$

where $K = K(k)$ is the complete elliptic integral of the first kind with the modulus k as a root of the **transcendental equation**

$$\frac{K(k')}{K(k)} = \frac{2b}{a}, \quad k' = \sqrt{1-k^2}, \quad 0 < k < 1. \tag{16}$$

Functions $\xi(x,y)$ and $\eta(x,y)$ are expressed in terms of Jacobian elliptic functions. Function $I(\xi,\eta)$ is an integral

$$I(\xi,\eta) = \int_0^1 \frac{\ln\left\{\left[\left(\frac{\sqrt{1-k'^2 t^2}}{k} - \xi\right)^2 + \eta^2\right]\left[\left(\frac{\sqrt{1-k'^2 t^2}}{k} + \xi\right)^2 + \eta^2\right]\right\}}{\sqrt{(1-t^2)(1-k'^2 t^2)}} \, dt. \tag{17}$$

which in some cases can be expressed in finite form, and

$$J_i^* = \begin{cases} J_i & \text{for capillary of the type } i = 1 \text{ in Fig. } 11 \\ 0.5\ J_i & \text{for capillary of the type } i = 2 \text{ in Fig. } 11 \\ 0.25\ J_i & \text{for capillary of the type } i = 3 \text{ or } 4 \text{ in Fig. } 11 \end{cases} \qquad (18)$$

The use of the boundary conditions yields linear relationships between the intracapillary oxygen tensions P_i and the diffusion fluxes J_j :

$$P_i = \frac{Ma_i}{D\alpha} - \frac{1}{D\alpha} \sum_{j=1}^{n} b_{ij}\ J_j + \nu P_o \qquad (19)$$

where the coefficients a_i, b_{ij} can be expressed in terms of the capillary coordinates (x_i, y_i); $\nu = \alpha/\alpha_b$. In addition, the conservation of mass of oxygen yields a constraint

$$\sum_{i=1}^{n} J_i^* = 4abM . \qquad (20)$$

Linear relationships (19), (20) can be resolved to express J_i and P_o as linear functions of P_i. Substitution of these relationships into equation (12) reduces the problem to the solution of a set of n nonlinear ordinary differential equations with appropriate boundary conditions.

As an example of calculations of this kind, we consider the case of a pair of capillaries located in the opposite corners of a parallelepiped. The inlets and outlets of the capillaries are located on the same planes so that the flow conditions are either concurrent or countercurrent. Typical parameters have been chosen for the skeletal muscle microcirculation. Fig. 12 shows variation of the mean PO_2 in the tissue, P_m, the minimum oxygen tension, P_{min} , and the PO_2 at the venous end of the capillary, P_v, with variation of the capillary velocity v for concurrent and countercurrent flow conditions. For comparison, the corresponding values obtained within the framework of the Krogh cylinder model are also shown.

In conclusion, it is appropriate to point out the factors and phenomena that may be of importance, at least in certain situations, and therefore, deserve further careful consideration. These are: spatial heterogeneity of the oxygen consumption, e.g. in mixed skeletal muscle in different types of fibers, as well as specific geometry of the capillary structure in relation to fibers; capillary anastomoses could undoubtedly play a role in tissue oxygenation, however, an adequate mathematical approach to this problem has yet to be developed; diffusional interaction between the tissue surface and capillary structures situated in the vicinity of the surface may be of importance, especially under experimental conditions. The role of these

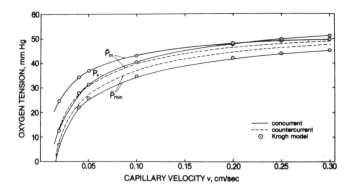

FIG. *12*. Variation of oxygen tensions with capillary velocity.

factors, as well as the factors considered previously within the
framework of the Krogh cylinder concept, such as the finite
resistivity of the capillary wall and vascular plasma layers to
oxygen diffusion, and the oxygen binding kinetics (10) ought to
be examined in future analyses of oxygen exchange between
capillary networks and the surrounding tissue.

ACKNOWLEDGMENTS

This work was supported by National Institutes of Health
Grants HL-23362 and HL-17421. The author wishes to thank
Dr. Bruce Klitzman for reading the manuscript and making critical
comments, and Ms. Gayle G. Caulton and Mrs. Mildred A. Long for
secretarial assistance.

REFERENCES

1. Aroesty, J., and Gross, J.F. (1970): Convection and diffu-
    sion in the microcirculation. Microvasc. Res., 2:247-267.

2. Bailey, H.R. (1967): Oxygen exchange between capillary and
    tissue: some equations describing countercurrent and non-
    linear transport. In: Physical Bases of Circulatory
    Transport. Regulation and Exchange, edited by E.B. Reeve,
    and A.C. Guyton, pp. 353-366. Saunders, Philadelphia.

3. Bugliarello, G., and Hsiao, C.C. (1964): Phase separation
    in suspension flowing through bifurcations: A simplified
    hemodynamic model. Science, 143:469-471.

4. Burton, K.S., and Johnson, P.C. (1972): Reactive hyperemia
    in individual capillaries of skeletal muscle. Am. J.
    Physiol. 223:517-524.

5. Cokelet, G.R. (1976): Macroscopic rheology and tube flow

of human blood. In: Microcirculation 1, edited by
J. Grayson, and W. Zingg, pp. 9-31, Plenum Press, New York.

6. Cokelet, G.R. (1978): Hemodynamics, In: Peripheral
Circulation, edited by P.C. Johnson, pp. 81-110, Wiley,
New York.

7. Diemer, K. (1963): Eine verbesserte Modellvorstellung zur
O_2-Versorgung des Gehirns. Naturwissenschaften, 50:617-618.

8. Duling, B.R., and Berne, R.M. (1970): Longitudinal gradients in periarteriolar oxygen tension. A possible mechanism for the participation of oxygen in local regulation of
blood flow. Circ. Res., 27:669-678.

9. Duling, B.R. and Pittman, R.N. (1975): Oxygen tension:
dependent or independent variable in local control of blood
flow. Fed. Proc., 34:2012-2019.

10. Fletcher, J.E. (1978): Mathematical modeling of the microcirculation. Math. Biosci., 38:159-202.

11. Fronek, K., and Zweifach, B.W. (1977): Microvascular blood
flow in cat tenuissimus muscle. Microvasc. Res., 14:
181-189.

12. Fung, Y.C. (1973): Stochastic flow in capillary blood
vessels. Microvasc. Res., 5:34-48.

13. Gaehtgens, P., Schmid-Schönbein, H., Schmidt, F., Will, G.
and Stöhr-Liesen, M. (1979): Comparative microrheology of
nucleated avian (NRBC) and non-nucleated human (HRBC)
erythrocytes during viscometric and small tube flow. 2nd
World Congress for Microcirculation, July 23-27, 1979,
La Jolla, CA., U.S.A., Abstracts Part II, pp. 53-54.

14. Gray, S.D., and Renkin, E.M. (1978): Microvascular supply
in relation to fiber metabolic type in mixed skeletal muscle
of rabbits. Microvasc. Res., 16:406-425.

15. Gross, J.F., Intaglietta, M., and Zweifach, B.W. (1974):
Network model of pulsatile hemodynamics in the microcirculation of the rabbit omentum. Am. J. Physiol., 226:1117-1123.

16. Grunewald, W.A. (1968): Theoretical analysis of the oxygen
supply in tissue. In: Oxygen Transport in Blood and Tissue,
edited by D.W. Lubbers et al., pp. 110-114, Thieme, Stuttgart.

17. Grunewald, W.A., and Sowa, W. (1977): Capillary structures
and O_2 supply to tissue. An analysis with a digital diffusion model as applied to the skeletal muscle. Rev. Physiol.
Biochem. Pharmacol. 77:149-209.

18. Grunewald, W.A., and Sowa, W. (1978): Distribution of the miocardial tissue PO_2 in the rat and the inhomogeneity of the coronary bed. Pflügers. Arch., 374:57-66.

19. Honig, C.R. (1977): Hypoxia in skeletal muscle at rest and during the transition to steady work. Microvasc. Res., 13:377-398.

20. Honig, C.R., Frierson, J.L., and Nelson, C.N. (1971): O_2 transport and VO_2 in resting muscle: significance for tissue - capillary exchange. Am. J. Physiol. 220:357-363.

21. Honig, C.R., Feldstein, M.L., and Frierson, J.L. (1977): Capillary lengths, anastomoses, and estimated capillary transit times in skeletal muscle. Am. J. Physiol., 233:122-129.

22. Johnson, P.C. (1971): Red cell separation in the mesenteric capillary network. Am. J. Physiol., 221:99-104.

23. Klabunde, R.E. and Johnson, P.C. (1977): Reactive hyperemia in capillaries of red and white skeletal muscle. Am. J. Physiol., 232:H411-H417.

24. Klitzman, B., and Duling, B.R. (1979): Microvascular hematocrit and red cell flow in resting and contracting striated muscle. Am J. Physiol., 237:H481-H490.

25. Krogh, A. (1919): The supply of oxygen to the tissues and the regulation of the capillary circulation. J. Physiol. (London), 52:457-474.

26. Kunze, K. (1969): Das Sauerstoffdruckfeld im normalen und pathologische veräderten Muskel. Schriftenreihe Neurologie, 3:1-118.

27. Lee, J.S. (1977): Pressure - flow relationships of single vessels and organs. In: Microcirculation, Vol. 1, edited by G. Kaley, and B.M. Altura, pp. 335-364. University Park Press, Baltimore.

28. Lee, J.S., and Nellis, S. (1974): Modeling study on the distribution of flow and volume in the microcirculation of cat mesentery. Annals Biomed. Eng., 2:206-216.

29. Leonard, E.F., and Jorgensen, S.B. (1974): The analysis of convection and diffusion in capillary beds. Annual Rev. Biophys. Bioeng., 3:293-339.

30. Lipowsky, H.H., and Zweifach, B.W. (1974): Network analysis of microcirculation of cat mesentery. Microvasc. Res., 7:73-83.

31. Lipowsky, H.H., and Zweifach, B.W. (1977): Methods for the simultaneous measurement of pressure differentials and flow in single unbranched vessels of the microcirculation for rheological studies. Microvasc. Res., 14:345-361.

32. Lipowsky, H.H., Kovalcheck, S., and Zweifach, B.W. (1978): The distribution of blood rheological parameters in the microvasculature of cat mesentery. Circ. Res., 43:738-749.

33. Lipowsky, H.H., Usami, S., and Chien, S. (1979): In vivo measurements of "apparent viscosity" and microvessel hematocrit in the mesentery of the cat. Microvasc. Res., (in press).

34. Mayrovitz, H.N., Wiedeman, M.P., and Noordergraaf, A. (1975): Microvascular hemodynamic variations accompanying microvessel dimensional changes. Microvasc. Res., 10: 322-339.

35. Mayrovitz, H.N., Wiedeman, M.P., and Nordergraff, A. (1976): Analytical characterization of microvascular resistance distribution. Bull. Math. Biol., 38:71-82.

36. Mayrovitz, H.N., Tuma, R.F., and Wiedeman, M.P. (1977): Relationship between microvascular blood velocity and pressure distribution. Am. J. Physiol., 232:H400-H405.

37. Mayrovitz, H.N., Wiedeman, M.P., and Noordergraaf, A., (1978): Interaction in the microcirculation. In: Cardiovascular System Dynamics, edited by J. Baan, A. Noordergraaf, and J. Raines, pp. 194-204. MIT Press, Cambridge, Massachusetts.

38. Metzger, H. (1969): Distribution of oxygen partial pressure in a two-dimensional tissue supplied by capillary meshes and concurrent and countercurrent systems. Math. Biosci., 5:143-154.

39. Metzger, H. (1973): Geometric considerations in modeling oxygen transport processes in tissue. Advances Exp. Med. Biol., 37b:761-772.

40. Metzger, H. (1976): The influence of space-distributed parameters on the calculation of substrate and gas exchange in microvascular units. Math. Biosci., 30:31-45.

41. Myrhage, R. (1977): Microvascular supply of skeletal muscle fibers. Acta Orthopaedica Scand. Suppl. 168:1-46.

42. Palmer, A.A., and Betts, W.H. (1975): The axial drift of
     fresh and acetaldehyde - hardened erythrocytes in 25μm
     capillary slits of various lengths. Biorheology, 12:
     282-292.

43. Pittman, R.N., and Duling, B.R. (1977): Effect of altered
     carbon dioxide tension on hemoglobin oxygenation in hamster
     cheek pouch microvessels. Microvasc. Res., 13:211-224.

44. Pittman, R.N., and Duling, B.R. (1977): The determination
     of oxygen availability in the microcirculation. In:
     Oxygen and Physiological Function, edited by F.F. Jöbsis,
     pp. 133-147. Professional Information Library, Dallas.

45. Popel, A.S. (1978): Analysis of capillary - tissue diffusion
     in multicapillary systems. Math. Biosci., 39:187-211.

46. Popel, A.S. (1979): Effect of heterogeneity of capillary
     flow on the capillary hematocrit. In: 1979 Biomechanics
     Symposium, edited by W.C. Van Buskirk, pp. 83-84. Amer.
     Soc. Mech. Eng., New York.

47. Popel, A.S. (1979): A model of pressure and flow distri-
     bution in branching networks. J. Appl. Mech. (in press).

48. Popel, A.S., and Gross, J.F. (1979): Analysis of oxygen
     diffusion from arteriolar networks. Am. J. Physiol.,
     237: (in press).

49. Reneau, D.D., and Knisely, M.H. (1971): A mathematical
     simulation of oxygen transport in the human brain under
     conditions of countercurrent capillary blood flow. Chem.
     Eng. Progr., 67:18-27.

50. Schmid-Schöenbein, G.W., and Zweifach, B.W. (1975): RBC
     velocity profiles in arterioles and venules of the rabbit
     omentum. Microvasc. Res., 10:153-164.

51. Schmid-Schöenbein, G.W., Skalak, R., Usami, S., and Chien, S.
     (1979): Cell distribution in capillary networks. Microvasc.
     Res. (in press).

52. Schmid-Schöenbein, H. and Devendran, Th. (1972): Blood
     rheology in the microcirculation. Pflügers Arch. (Suppl.),
     336:84.

53. Schmid-Schoenbein, H. (1976): Microrheology of erythrocytes,
     blood viscosity, and the distribution of blood flow in the
     microcirculation. In: Cardiovascular Physiology II, Vol. 9,
     edited by A.C. Guyton and A.W. Cowley, pp. 1-62, University
     Park Press, Baltimore.

54. Vaupel, P., Grunewald, W.A., Manz, R., and Sowa, W. (1978):
     Intracapillary HbO_2 saturation in tumor tissue of DS-
     carcinosarcoma during normoxia. Advances Exp. Med. Biol.,
     94:367-375.

55. Wiedeman, M. (1963): Dimensions of blood vessels from
     distributing artery to collecting vein. Circ. Res., 12:
     375-378.

56. Yen, R.T., and Fung, Y.C. (1978): Effect of velocity
     distribution on red cell distribution in capillary blood
     vessels. Am. J. Physiol., 235:H251-H257.

Mathematics of Microcirculation Phenomena,
edited by J. F. Gross and A. Popel.
Raven Press, New York © 1980.

Convection and Diffusion in the Extravascular Space

Eric P. Salathé

*Center for the Application of Mathematics, Lehigh University,
Bethlehem, Pennsylvania 18015*

INTRODUCTION

The increase in blood pressure required to supply nutrients and oxygen to tissue in higher forms of life is accompanied by an increase in concentration of plasma protein. The resulting osmotic pressure prevents excessive escape of fluid from the capillaries that would otherwise occur due to hydrostatic pressure. The capillary endothelium may be regarded as a porous membrane freely permeable to water but relatively impermeable to the large protein molecules. Starling hypothesized that the direction and rate of flow of fluid across the capillary membrane is proportional to the sum of the hydrostatic and protein osmotic pressure differences. This was confirmed by Landis [5] through direct measurements on single capillaries in the mesentery of the frog.

While the osmotic pressure of the plasma proteins is fairly constant, the hydrostatic pressure varies not only in time, but also along the length of the capillary at any fixed time. Measurements by Landis show that the combined pressure effect may favor reabsorption of fluid at the venous end of the capillary. However, in some tissues, in certain cases, an excess of filtration over reabsorption occurs and there is a net filtration of fluid into the surrounding tissue. In addition, there is a steady leakage of plasma proteins through the capillary walls, and in the course of a day approximately 50% of the total circulating protein escapes from the blood vessels. An extensive review of the exchange of substances across capillary walls has been given by Landis and Pappenheimer [6].

The plasma proteins which escape from the blood vessels cannot be reabsorbed into the capillaries. The mechanism by which escaped plasma proteins as well as the net fluid which enters the tissue is returned to the blood stream is found in the lymphatic system. The lymphatic vessels form a fine network of thin walled capillaries which combine into large collecting ducts. These ducts return the lymph to the blood stream, mainly by way of the large veins at the base of the neck, although other lymphatic-venous connections exist. The escaped plasma proteins together with unabsorbed tissue fluid readily enter the lymph capillaries and so are returned to the blood stream indirectly. The total amount of lymph flow is not known with certainty, but the available evidence suggests that in 24 hours the thoracic duct alone returns to the blood stream a quantity of lymph approximately equal to the blood volume. A comprehensive description of the lymphatic system has been provided by Yoffey and Courtice [14].

Spacial variation in interstitial fluid hydrostatic and osmotic pressures occur as a result of capillary-tissue exchange. For example, gradients in interstitial hydrostatic pressure must exist in order to move the filtered or reabsorbed fluid either away from or toward the capillary. Along a section of capillary that is filtering, the pericapillary protein concentration is diluted as a result of the fluid entering the interstitial space. Similarly, during reabsorption the moving interstitial fluid convects interstitial protein toward the capillary. These proteins cannot enter the capillary, and so they accumulate in the adjacent tissue. The resulting arterial-venous pericapillary osmotic pressure gradient is further enhanced by plasma protein leakage, since experimental evidence suggests that such leakage is greater at the venous end of the capillary.

Under normal circumstances, fluid exchange is so small relative to capillary flow that the plasma protein concentration is effectively constant along the length of the capillary. However, under certain pathological conditions excessive filtration occurs and a significant axial gradient in plasma protein concentration results. Under such conditions the hydrostatic pressure variation within the capillary is also affected.

Many small molecules and ions delivered to the tissue by blood, such as glucose, or removed from the tissue by blood, such as lactate, contribute an osmotic pressure difference across the capillary wall and Starling's law must be generalized to take their effect into account. Since the capillary is fairly permeable to these substances, the osmotic effect must be computed by introducing a reflection coefficient for each species. The concentration of each substance must be determined through an analysis of their convection and diffusion in the capillary and in the surrounding tissue. Such analysis must consider the mechanisms by which transport across the capillary wall occurs. These mechanisms include simple or facilitated diffusion, solvent drag, or active transport, and may involve a saturation phenomenon in which no additional transport takes place when a limiting concentration is reached.

Since the various pressures involved in Starling's law are affected by filtration and reabsorption, it is clear that capillary-tissue fluid exchange represents a complex coupling of the flow and diffusion processes within the capillary and in the surrounding interstitial space.

The microcirculation is a dynamic system, with blood flow continuously being altered as regulating arterioles and precapillary sphincters open and close to meet the changing metabolic needs of the tissue. The large drop in capillary pressure that results when an arteriole or sphincter contracts can cause a capillary to change from a condition of filtration to one of reabsorption. Since the reabsorbed fluid enters the capillary during a period of reduced flow velocity, the interluminal protein concentration may be sufficiently diluted that the driving force for reabsorption is substantially diminished. The affect of such time dependent processes on the interstitial fluid pressure and protein concentration can only be determined through an analysis of the full unsteady equations governing these quantities.

Additional unsteady effects occur as a result of transient hypertonicity in the tissue. The rapid outpouring of fluid from the capillaries following burn injury, or the increased filtration that occurs to meet the elevated metabolic requirements of cells during exercise, is a result of small ions and particles in the tissue. The increased filtration persists until production of these metabolites ceases and they are washed away by the capillary blood flow.

In the following sections a theory of interstitial fluid movement and protein transport will be derived and incorporated into a model of capillary-tissue fluid exchange. The formulation will be sufficiently general to include all of the phenomena outlined above. In subsequent sections, various analytic techniques for solving these equations will be described, and the solution to a number of different problems discussed.

FLUID AND PROTEIN MOVEMENT IN THE INTERSTITIAL SPACE

The water, protein, and particles that are exchanged between blood capillaries and the surrounding tissue move through the small interstitial spaces between the cells. An understanding of interstitial fluid motion and the convection and diffusion of particles in the interstitial space is essential to the study of capillary exchange and blood-lymph transport. The interstitial space is a two-phase system, consisting of a gel-like phase and a free-fluid phase, in which the free fluid is distributed between the cells in a thin layer of less than 1 µm . McMaster [7] observed that over a range of pressures from 4.5 to 14 cm H_2O the entry of fluid into the tissue through a needle was slow and intermittent, but at pressures greater than 14 cm H_2O , which he termed the breaking point, fluid flowed at a much more rapid rate. Guyton, Scheel and Murphree [4] measured the rate of fluid movement between two perforated catheters inserted into the tissue. Fluid movement between the catheters increased as the mean pressure level was raised, even though the pressure difference between the catheters remained fixed. Resistance to fluid motion was very high at normal tissue pressure, but when a certain critical pressure was exceeded, the resistance decreased more than 100,000-fold. This critical pressure is analogous to McMaster's breaking point and was determined by Guyton to occur at atmospheric pressure.

The structure of interstitial space and the experimental evidence suggest that interstitial fluid moves as a result of a gradient of interstitial fluid pressure and can be described in a manner analogous to flow through a porous medium, although with some significant differences. In an earlier paper [9], the interstitial fluid velocity, $\underset{\sim}{v}$, and pressure, p , were related by a generalized form of Darcy's law, $\underset{\sim}{v} = - K_t(p)\underset{\sim}{\nabla}p$ where the hydrodynamic conductivity of the tissue, K_t , was assumed to be a function of the pressure. The form of this function was later determined [1] from the experiments of Guyton, Scheel and Murphree.

Although there is a paucity of interstitial fluid under normal conditions, free fluid in pools has been observed during edema, and the increase in interstitial fluid volume is accompanied by an increase in tissue pressure. Using a tissue osmometer, Wiederhielm [12] obtained a relationship between tissue swelling pressure and volume; Guyton [3] measured interstitial fluid pressure from implanted perforated capsules while varying interstitial volume. In both cases it was found that at low pressure considerable increase in pressure is required to increase fluid volume, but at higher pressures the compliance of the tissue increases significantly. The volume flow rate of interstitial fluid, q , is related to the interstitial fluid velocity by $q = \theta v$, where θ is the porosity of the tissue, or the fraction of a given portion of tissue occupied by mobile interstitial fluid. The porosity is also a function of the interstitial fluid pressure, and the form of this function, $\theta(p)$, can be determined from experimental results [1].

The principle of conservation of mass requires that the net fluid flux from any given volume of tissue must equal the rate of decrease in the quantity of fluid contained in that portion of tissue. Since the porosity, θ , represents the fraction of tissue occupied by mobile interstitial fluid, this principle is expressed by $\partial\theta/\partial t + \underset{\sim}{\nabla}\cdot q = 0$. Therefore, the fundamental equation for the interstitial fluid pressure is

$$\frac{\partial}{\partial t}\,\theta(p) - \underset{\sim}{\nabla}\cdot\theta(p)K_t(p)\underset{\sim}{\nabla}p = 0 \ . \tag{1}$$

For steady flow this reduces to $\underset{\sim}{\nabla}\cdot\theta K_t\underset{\sim}{\nabla}p = 0$, and for θ , K_t constant, to Laplace's equation, $\underset{\sim}{\nabla}^2p = 0$.

Extravascular protein moves through interstitial space as a result of diffusion and of convection by the moving interstitial fluid. The diffusion velocity of protein is proportional to the gradient of concentration, c , and is given by $\underset{\sim}{U} = - D\underset{\sim}{\nabla}c$, where D is the diffusion coefficient. For diffusion in an unbounded fluid D would be the free diffusion coefficient. However, for proteins moving in the small pores occupied by the interstitial fluid significant deviation from the free diffusion coefficient will occur, and a strong dependence of D on the pore size may be expected. The diffusion coefficient must be regarded as a function of porosity θ , and therefore, of interstitial fluid pressure p . The nature of the function D(p) must be determined experimentally. In the absence of diffusion, protein is still transported by the motion of the interstitial fluid. In an unbounded fluid the velocity of transport would be the fluid

velocity, but in the small channels through which interstitial
fluid moves there are significant wall effects and it is to be
expected that the convection velocity, V , will differ from
the interstitial fluid velocity v . This can be expressed by
writing $V = \lambda v$, where the factor λ $(0 \leq \lambda \leq 1)$ will, in general,
depend on the size of the channels, and consequently on the inter-
stitial fluid pressure. Therefore $\lambda = \lambda(p)$ must also be regarded as an arbitrary but known function to be determined experimentally. The flux of protein per unit area of tissue is
$q^* = \theta(cV+U)$. Since conservation of protein requires
$\partial/\partial t \; \theta c + \tilde{\nabla} \cdot q^* = 0$, the governing equation for extravascular protein concentration c is

$$\frac{\partial}{\partial t} \theta(p)c + \nabla \cdot [c\lambda(p)\theta(p)K_t(p)\nabla p + \theta(p)D(p)\nabla c] = 0 . \qquad (2)$$

MATHEMATICAL THEORY OF CAPILLARY-TISSUE EXCHANGE

As a result of capillary-tissue exchange, the hydrostatic pressure and the concentration of protein and diffusible materials,
both in the capillary and in the adjacent tissue, vary with time
and position. If the distance between capillaries is sufficiently
large, the disturbances in the tissue surrounding a capillary decay to a uniform background value without interacting with the
disturbances surrounding an adjacent capillary. Previous studies
[1], [9] show that a capillary spacing of the order of half the
capillary length is sufficient for this to be the case. When this
criterion is satisfied, direct interaction between capillaries
does not occur and an appropriate model consists of a single capillary surrounded by an infinite tissue. Far from the capillary
the interstitial pressure and the concentration of protein and
other diffusible substances have uniform values. The actual
values specified depend on the nature of the entire capillary bed,
including the effect of any lymphatics present, and so represents
the indirect interaction of the various capillaries.

The model, therefore, consists of a simple straight circular
capillary of length L and radius R_c , exchanging fluid and substances with the surrounding tissue. Blood enters the capillary
at the arterial end with known pressure P_A . In addition, either
the rate of blood flow entering the capillary, Q_O , or the pressure at the venous end, P_V , must be specified. In general, these
three quantities are functions of time.

Fluid exchange occurs as a result of the combined hydrostatic
and osmotic pressure differences across the capillary wall. The
hydrostatic and osmotic pressures of the plasma, P and Π ,
respectively, are assumed to be functions only of distance z
along the capillary, since any variation across the capillary is
negligible. The interstitial hydrostatic and osmotic pressures,
p and π , respectively, depend not only on z , but also on distance r normal to the capillary axis. Fluid exchange is governed by Starling's law,

$$\text{F.M.} = k_f(z)[P(z) - p(R_c,z) + \pi(R_c,z) - \Pi(z)] \qquad 0 \leq z \leq L \qquad (3)$$

where F.M. is the volume rate of fluid movement per unit area of capillary wall (+, filtration; -, reabsorption), and k_f is the filtration coefficient. In general, k_f varies with distance along the capillary and can increase as much as 10-fold from the arterial to the venous end. In eqn. (3), the interstitial pressures π and p are evaluated at the capillary wall, $r = R_c$.

Starling's law, eqn. (3), can be generalized to include the osmotic effect of various diffusible substances in the microcirculation. If C_i and c_i represent the concentration of the i'th species, $i = 1-n$, in the capillary and in the tissue, respectively, and Π_i and π_i the corresponding osmotic pressures, each species contributes an osmotic effect given by $\sigma_i(z)[\pi_i(R_c,z)-\Pi_i(z)]$, where $\sigma_i (0<\sigma_i<1)$ is the corresponding reflection coefficient. Since the permeability generally varies along the length of the capillary, increasing from the arterial to the venous end, the reflection coefficients must be regarded as functions of z . The species concentration in the capillary is also assumed to vary only with axial position, radial variation being ignored. The justification for this lies in the nature of the capillary flow. The red blood cells travel single file through the capillary, separated by a bolus of fluid in which the plasma undergoes a recirculating, eddy-like motion. The resultant convective mixing causes a fairly uniform radial concentration profile. The generalized form of Starling's law is then

$$\text{F.M.} = k_f(z)\{P(z) - p(R_c,z) + \sigma(z)[\pi(R_c,z) - \Pi(z)]$$
$$+ \sum_{i=1}^{n} \sigma_i(z)[\pi_i(R_c,z) - \Pi_i(z)]\} \ . \qquad (4)$$

A reflection coefficient for the protein osmotic pressure, $\sigma(z)$, has been included in this generalization, since the capillary wall is not ideally semi-permeable to protein. The osmotic pressures are determined from the protein concentrations. Both plasma and interstitial fluid show significant deviation from van't Hoff's law, but the osmotic pressure can be accurately represented by a third order polynomial in concentration. The general theory, however, may be developed in terms of the arbitrary functional dependences $\Pi = H(C)$, $\pi = h(c)$, $\Pi_i = H_i(C_i)$, $\pi_i = h_i(C_i)$, with definite functions assumed only when specific numerical examples are considered.

Flow within the capillary is governed by a generalized form of Poiseuille's law,

$$Q = - \frac{\pi}{8\mu}[R_c(z)]^4 \frac{dP}{dz} , \qquad (5)$$

which states that the volume flow rate of blood through the

capillary, $Q(z)$, is proportional to the local pressure gradient, dP/dz . An apparent viscosity, μ , is used to account for the effect of red blood cells [9]. The capillary radius is assumed to be a function of z , since in some tissue it increases from the arterial to the venous end.

Protein concentration within the capillary changes not only as a result of direct protein leakage, but also as a result of fluid exchange with the surrounding tissue. A mass balance equation for protein inside a small length, Δz , of the capillary yields the equation

$$\frac{\partial C}{\partial t} + \frac{1}{\pi R_c^2} \frac{d}{dz} QC = -(\frac{2}{R_c}) \text{ P.L.} \tag{6}$$

where P.L. represents the capillary-tissue protein loss per unit area of capillary wall. Axial diffusion of protein in the capillary has been neglected in obtaining this result.

The interstitial fluid pressure and protein concentration are governed by eqns. (1) and (2). To these must be added the one-dimensional water balance equation

$$\frac{dQ}{dz} = 2\pi R_c(z) \left[\theta(p) K_t(p) \frac{\partial p}{\partial r} \right]_{r=R_c} , \tag{7}$$

which relates the change in volume flow rate to fluid exchange, and the boundary condition for interstitial protein flux at the capillary wall,

$$\left[-\theta D \frac{\partial c}{\partial r} - \lambda c \theta K_t \frac{\partial p}{\partial r} \right]_{r=R_c} = \text{P.L.} \tag{8}$$

This last equation states that the rate of convection and diffusion of protein away from the capillary at the wall equals the rate of protein loss per unit area.

The diffusion of the small, osmotically active metabolites included in the generalization of Starling's law is so rapid that their convection by the interstitial fluid can be neglected. Their concentration in the tissue is therefore governed by the equations

$$\frac{\partial}{\partial t} \theta c_i + \nabla \cdot \theta D_i \nabla c_i = 0 , \tag{9}$$

where D_i is the diffusion coefficient of the i'th metabolite. Species conservation in the capillary gives an equation analogous to eqns. (6) and (8) for protein:

$$\frac{\partial C_i}{\partial t} + \frac{1}{\pi R_c^2} \frac{d}{dz} QC_i = -\frac{2}{R_c} \alpha_i(z) [C_i - c_i] = \frac{2}{R_c} \left[\theta D_i \frac{\partial c_i}{\partial r} \right]_{R_c} \tag{10}$$

where it has been assumed that capillary-tissue flux is proportional to the concentration difference across the capillary wall.

The permeability coefficient for each species, α_i , is assumed to be a known function of distance along the capillary.

The mathematical formulation is completed by specifying boundary and initial conditions. The specific conditions imposed depend on the particular problem being considered. For steady problems, this usually involves giving the uniform conditions in the interstitial space far from the capillary and in the arterial blood entering the capillary. This is expressed by the equations

$$p(r,z) \to p_\infty , \quad c(r,z) \to c_\infty , \quad c_i(r,z) \to c_{i\infty} \quad \text{as} \quad r^2+z^2 \to \infty ,$$
(11)

$$P(0) = P_A , \quad Q(0) = Q_o , \quad C(0) = C_A , \quad C_i(0) = C_{iA} .$$

Appropriate boundary and initial conditions for various time dependent problems will be discussed later.

NON-LINEAR STEADY PROBLEMS

In this section all pressures will be normalized by the arterial pressure P_A and the protein concentration by its value in the arterial blood, C_A . Distances will be normalized by the capillary length L and the hydrodynamic conductivity, tissue porosity, and protein diffusivity by their values in the tissue far from the capillary. The same notation will be used for these variables, but it is to be understood that they are normalized.

For time independent processes eqns. (1) and (2) reduce to

$$\nabla \cdot \theta(p) K_t(p) \nabla p = 0$$
(12)

$$\nabla \cdot [c\lambda(p)\theta(p)K_t(p)\nabla p] + \alpha\nabla \cdot [\theta(p)D(p)\nabla c] = 0 ,$$
(13)

where $\alpha = \hat{D}_\infty / \hat{K}_{t\infty} P_A$. ($\hat{D}_\infty$, $\hat{K}_{t\infty}$, as well as $\hat{\theta}_\infty$, refer to the dimensional value of these three quantities in the uniform region far from the capillary.) If a new variable, ϕ , is introduced, defined by $d\phi/dp = \theta(p)K_t(p)$, $\phi(p_\infty) = 0$, eqn. (12) reduces to Laplace's equation,

$$\nabla^2\phi = 0 .$$
(14)

A solution to eqn. (14) satisfying the condition $\phi \to 0$ as $r^2 + z^2 \to \infty$ can be expressed in terms of an arbitrary function $f(z)$, defined on the interval $0 \le z \le 1$, by

$$\phi = \int_o^1 \frac{f(\zeta)d\zeta}{\sqrt{(\zeta-z)^2+r^2}} .$$
(15)

Equation (15) states that the interstitial fluid pressure can be represented as a distribution of sources and sinks for the function ϕ distributed along the capillary axis, and reduces the determination of $p(r,z)$ to the determination of a function of only one variable, $f(z)$. It will be seen that positive f (sources) corresponds to filtration and negative f (sinks) corresponds to reabsorption. Note that when θ and K_t are constant, $\nabla^2 p = 0$ and ϕ can be replaced by $p-p_\infty$.

Equation (13) admits a solution of the form $c = F(\phi)$, which states that the interstitial protein concentration is a function only of the interstitial fluid pressure. This can be seen by substituting the assumption $c = F(\phi)$ into eqn. (13), which gives $(d/d\phi)(\alpha\theta DdF/d\phi+\lambda F) = 0$. Integrating this expression yields $\alpha\theta DdF/d\phi+\lambda F = $ constant. Since θ, D and λ are known functions of p , and therefore of ϕ , this last expression is indeed an equation for $F(\phi)$, which proves the conjecture. For such a solution to be possible however, it must be consistent not only with the governing equation for c , but also the related boundary conditions. In the present case, this is eqn. (8). Substituting $c = F(\phi)$ into the normalized form of eqn. (8) gives $\alpha\theta DdF/d\phi + \lambda F = P.L.(L/C_A\hat{\theta}_\infty\hat{K}_{t\infty}P_A)/[-\partial\phi/dr]_{r=R}$ where $R = R_c/L$. This is consistent with the above integral of the governing equation if and only if protein loss is proportional to fluid movement across the capillary wall, so that $P.L./[-d\phi/dr]_{r=R} = $ constant $(=\beta$, say). This is generally not the case, since, for example, it would imply that protein is convected into the capillary during reabsorption. However, in certain pathological cases, such as following capillary damage, fluid convection may be the principle transport mechanism for capillary-tissue protein transport and the above requirement would be satisfied. It then follows that

$$c = e^{-\frac{1}{\alpha}\int_0^\phi \frac{\lambda(\psi)}{\theta(\psi)D(\psi)} d\psi} \left\{ c_\infty + \beta \int_0^\phi e^{\frac{1}{\alpha}\int_0^\xi \frac{\lambda(\psi)}{\theta(\psi)D(\psi)} d\psi} d\xi \right\}. \quad (16)$$

For the special case $\beta = 0$ the above solution reduces to

$$c = c_\infty e^{-\frac{1}{\alpha}\int_0^\phi \frac{\lambda(\psi)}{\theta(\psi)D(\psi)} d\psi}. \quad (17)$$

This corresponds to neglecting leakage of protein across the capillary. Since such leakage is normally very small, it is a reasonable approximation. The disturbances to the extravascular protein distribution described by eqn. (17) are due entirely to the convective effect of the filtered and reabsorbed fluid. A better appreciation of the meaning of this solution can be attained by assuming λ , D and θ are constants. It then follows that $\phi = (p-p_\infty)$ and $c = c_\infty \exp[-(\hat{K}_{t\infty}P_A\lambda/\hat{D}_\infty)(p-p_\infty)]$. The deviation of c from c_∞ is therefore directly related to the deviation of p from p_∞ . The extravascular protein disturbance decreases with increasing $\hat{D}_\infty$ and with decreasing $\hat{K}_{t\infty}$

and λ , as would be expected. It also follows that $\partial p/\partial r$ and $\partial c/\partial r$ have opposite signs, so that during filtration protein concentration decreases from c_∞ as the capillary is approached, while during reabsorption the opposite is true.

If protein loss is neglected, plasma protein concentration varies only as a result of fluid exchange. From eqn. (6) and the boundary condition eqn. (11) it follows that the normalized concentration is $C(z) = Q_0/Q(z)$. Substituting $Q(z)$ from eqn. (5) gives the capillary protein concentration directly in terms of the capillary pressure:

$$C(z) = - \hat{Q}_0/[R(z)]^4 P'(z) , \qquad (18)$$

where $\hat{Q}_0 = (8\mu/\pi L^3 P_A)Q_0$.

The above results allow Starling's law, eqn. (3), to be written in the form

$$-\frac{\partial \phi}{\partial r}\bigg|_{r=R} = K(z)[P(z) - p(\phi(R,z)) + \bar{\pi}(\phi(R,z)) - \Pi(C(z))] \qquad (19)$$

where $\bar{\pi} = \bar{\pi}(\phi) = \pi[C(\phi)]$ is a known function of ϕ , and $K = Lk_f(z)/\hat{\theta}_\infty \hat{K}_{t\infty}$. Combining eqns. (5) and (7) gives

$$\frac{d}{dz}[R^4(z)\frac{dP}{dz}] = - A \ R(z)\frac{\partial \phi}{\partial r}\bigg|_{r=R} \qquad (20)$$

where $A = 16\mu\hat{\theta}_\infty \hat{K}_{t\infty}/L^2$. Since $C(z)$ has been determined in terms of $P(z)$, and ϕ in terms of $f(z)$, eqns. (19) and (20) represent two simultaneous equations for $P(z)$ and $f(z)$. The use of eqn. (15) for $\phi(R,z)$ and $\partial \phi/\partial R|_{r=R}$ in eqns. (19) and (20) can be considerably simplified by introducing the asymptotic expansions, valid for $R \ll 1$,

$$\phi(R,z) \sim -2f(z)\ln R + \int_0^1 \frac{f(\zeta)-f(z)}{|\zeta-z|} \, d\zeta$$

$$+ f(z)\ln[(4z)(1-z)] + O(R) \qquad (21)$$

$$\partial \phi/\partial r|_{r=R} \sim -2f(z)/R + O(R) . \qquad (22)$$

The leading terms in eqns. (21) and (22) (the $\ln R$ term in eqn. (21) and the $1/R$ terms in eqn. (22)) are the expressions for ϕ and $\partial \phi/\partial r$ due to a source in two dimensions, and involve the source strength f only at the local position z . The next order term in eqn. (21) (the order one term) involves the entire distribution of f over the length of the capillary in the determination of ϕ at any location z , and therefore includes the mutual interaction of the entire capillary. Unfortunately, the $\ln R$ term is not sufficiently large that the order one term can be neglected in comparison. (For example, if $R = 10^{-2}$, $|\ln R|$ is only about 4.6.) Although including terms to order one greatly increases the complexity of the solution, it is necessary to do so in order to obtain meaningful results. However, it is possible to use only the dominant term to obtain a first approximation and to include the order one term as a perturbation.

Even with $\phi = -2f \ln R$ and $\partial\phi/\partial r|_R = -2f/R$, eqns. (19) and (20) are still intractable. An additional simplification can be made, however, since filtration and reabsorption usually have only a small effect on the capillary pressure $P(z)$. Even under pathological cases when excessive filtration occurs, it is still possible to write this pressure in the form $P(z) = P_o(z) + P_1(z)$, where $P_o(z)$ is the capillary pressure that would pertain if no fluid exchange occurred, and P_1 is a small perturbation to this dominant term. The leading term, $P_o(z)$, is found from eqn. (20), neglecting fluid exchange, and is therefore given by

$$P_o(z) = 1 - \hat{Q}_o \int_o^z [R(\zeta)]^{-4} d\zeta . \tag{23}$$

With $P(z)$ now a known function, given approximately by $P_o(z)$, the dominant approximation for f, denoted by $f_o(z)$, is found from eqn. (19):

$$\frac{2f_o}{R} = K(z)\{P_o(z) - p(-2f_o \ln R) + \bar{\pi}(-2f_o \ln R) - \Pi(1)\} . \tag{24}$$

In this equation the plasma protein concentration remains constant as a result of the neglect of fluid exchange on $P(z)$ (c.f., eqn. (18)).

The effect of fluid exchange on $P(z)$ can be found by substituting $P(z) = P_o(z) + P_1(z)$ into eqn. (20) and using the approximate solution $f_o(z)$ to evaluate $\partial\phi/\partial r|_{r=R}$. Therefore $(d/dz[R^4 dP_1/dz] = 2Af_o(z)$. With the boundary conditions $P_1(0) = P_1'(0) = 0$, the solution is

$$P_1(z) = 2A \int_o^z \frac{d\zeta}{R^4(\zeta)} \int_o^z f_o(\zeta)d\zeta$$

$$- 2A \int_o^z f_o(\zeta)\left(\int_o^\zeta \frac{d\eta}{R^4(\eta)}\right)d\zeta . \tag{25}$$

The approximation $f_o(z)$ must be corrected to take into account the influence of fluid exchange on $P(z)$ and the influence of the $0(1)$ term in the expansion, eq. (21). This is done by writing $f \sim f_o(z) + f_1(z)$, where f_1 is a small perturbation to f_o. Substituting this expansion into eqn. (21) gives

$$\phi \sim -2f_o \ln R - 2f_1 \ln R + G(f_o) , \quad \text{where} \quad G(f) = \int_o^1 \{[f(\zeta)-f(z)]/$$

$|\zeta-z|\}d\zeta + f(z) \ln[4z(1-z)]$ is the $0(1)$ term. Therefore, $p(\phi) = p(-2f_o \ln R) + p'(-2f_o \ln R)[-2f_1 \ln R + G(f_o)]$, with a similar expansion for $\bar{\pi}(\phi)$. With $P(z) = P_o + P_1$ it follows from eqn. (18) that $C(z) \sim -\hat{Q}_o/[-\hat{Q}_o + R^4 P_1'] \sim 1 + [R(z)]^4 P_1'/\hat{Q}_o$, so that $\Pi(C) \sim \Pi(1) + \Pi'(1)[R(z)]^4 P_1'/\hat{Q}_o$ where $\Pi'(1)$ is $d\Pi/dC$ at $C=1$. Substituting these expansions and $P = P_o + P_1$ into eqn. (19) and making use of eqn. (24) gives

$$\frac{2f_1}{R} = K(z)\{P_1(z) + [p'(-2f_o \ln R)$$

$$- \bar{\pi}'(-2f_o \ln R)][2f_1 \ln R - G(f_o)]$$

$$= \Pi'(1)[R(z)]^4 P_1'/Q_o\} . \tag{26}$$

This can easily be solved explicitly for $f_1(z)$.

The expressions $P_o + P_1$, $f_o + f_1$, given by the above solutions, provide suitable approximations for P and f . The functions $R_c(z)$, $k_f(z)$, $K_t(p)$, $\theta(p)$, $D(p)$ and $\lambda(p)$ have been left completely general in obtaining these solutions. To obtain numerical results, each of these functions must be specified explicitly. A 50% increase in capillary diameter has been observed in some tissue, and since the radius appears to the fourth power, this has a significant effect on the capillary pressure [2]. Studies of the variation in the filtration coefficient along the length of the capillary have been reported by a number of authors. In intestinal capillaries k_f can increase by as much as 10 fold from the arterial to the venous end. The dependence of θ and K_t on p can be represented by [1] $\theta = \{1+(1/c-1)\exp[-aP_A(p-\hat{p})]\}^{-1}$ and $\theta K_t = B\exp(bP_A p)$ where $\hat{p}$ is normal tissue pressure. Good agreement with experimental results is attained for $a = 0.32$ mmHg^{-1} and $b = 2.2$ mmHg^{-1} [1], [10]. The constant B is found from $B = \theta(\hat{p})K_t(\hat{p})\exp(-bP_A\hat{p})$. Since there is no data available for $\theta(\hat{p})K_t(\hat{p})$, its value can be estimated to be $N k_f \Delta x/\theta_\infty K_{t\infty}$, where Δx is the capillary wall thickness. This implies that the tissue is N times more permeable than a corresponding thickness of capillary endothelium. Values of N from 50 to 500 have been employed [1], [8]. There does not appear to be any experimental studies from which to determine the functions $D(p)$ and $\lambda(p)$. However, some measurements of D have been reported for various tissues, and these can be used with the simplification D = constant to provide typical values.

Various special cases of the solutions obtained here have been described previously [1], [2], [9], [10] for a wide variety of physiological situations. The disturbances to interstitial fluid pressure and protein concentration caused by fluid exchange extend for a distance of several hundred microns into the tissue. At the capillary wall, the pressure can differ by several millimeters of mercury from its value far from the capillary, depending on the magnitude of the capillary filtration coefficient and the hydrodynamic conductivity. Using a physiologically reasonable value of 10^{-11} m^2/s for protein diffusivity, D , it was found that significant washout or accumulation of interstitial protein occurred as a result of filtration or reabsorption, respectively. Filtration is aided by the dependence of θ and K_t on p , since the increased pericapillary interstitial fluid pressure results in greater mobility of the interstitial fluid. The

reverse is true for reabsorption, and a limit exists on the
amount of fluid that can be reabsorbed into the capillary, since
tissue mobility approaches zero as the pericapillary interstitial
fluid pressure decreases. For given arterial pressure and blood
flow rate, an increase in capillary radius produces a higher
venous pressure than for a capillary with constant radius, resulting in a decreased driving force for filtration. This is
somewhat compensated for by the increased filtration coefficient
at the venous end. All these effects interact in a complex
manner, but their influence on capillary-tissue exchange can be
examined by means of the analytic solutions presented here.

LINEAR STEADY PROBLEMS

Although the solutions obtained in the previous section are
very general in the sense that they include arbitrary functional
dependence of R and k_f on z and of θ, K_t, λ and D, on
p, they neglect the effect of the osmotically active diffusible
metabolites, such as glucose and lactate, and neglect protein loss
from the capillary. In this section solutions will be obtained
that include these effects.

When θ and K_t are constant, eqn. (1) reduces to Laplace's
equation, $\nabla^2 p = 0$, for the normalized interstitial fluid pressure p. If it is assumed that protein movement through the
interstitial space is entirely due to diffusion, then the interstitial protein concentration c and the interstitial concentration of each diffusible metabolite c_i are also governed by
Laplace's equation $\nabla^2 c = 0$, $\nabla^2 c_i = 0$, provided their diffu-
sivities are constant. These concentrations are all assumed to be
normalized by their concentration in the arterial blood, so that
c and c_i are nondimensional quantities. In the remainder of
this section, the protein concentration will not be considered
separately, but will be regarded as one of the concentrations
c_i, i = 1-n. If p_∞ and $c_{i\infty}$ denote the normalized pressure
and concentrations far from the capillary, it follows, in a
manner analogous to eqn. (15), that

$$p = p_\infty + \int_0^1 \frac{f(\zeta)d\zeta}{\sqrt{(\zeta-z)^2+r^2}} \quad , \quad c_i = c_{i\infty} + \int_0^1 \frac{g_i(\zeta)d\zeta}{\sqrt{(\zeta-z)^2+r^2}} \quad , \quad (27)$$

and that at the capillary wall asymptotic representations of the
form given by eqns. (21) and (22) hold.

Substituting these results into the generalized form of
Starling's law, eqn. (4), and using eqns. (5) and (8) gives, for
constant capillary radius,

$$\frac{2}{R} f(z) = K(z)\{P(z) - p_\infty + 2f(z)\ln R + G(f)$$

$$+ \sum_{i=1}^{n} \beta_i \sigma_i(z)[c_{i\infty} - 2g_i \ln R + G(g_i) - C_i(z)]\} = A \frac{d^2P}{dz^2} \quad , \quad (28)$$

where linear relationships $\pi_i = \beta_i C_i$, $\Pi_i = \beta_i C_i$, have been

assumed between the normalized concentrations and their corresponding osmotic pressures.

Substituting the asymptotic expansions for c_i and $\partial c_i / \partial r$
into the normalized form of eqn. (10), and making use of eqn. (5)
for Q , gives

$$\frac{2}{R} g_i(z) = a_i(z)[C_i(z) - c_{i\infty} + 2g_i \ln R - G(g_i)] = \gamma \frac{d}{dz}[C_i \frac{dP}{dz}] \quad (29)$$

where $\gamma = R_c^3 P_A / 16\mu LD$ and $a_i(z) = (L/D)\alpha_i(z)$.

Equations (28), (29) represent $2(n+1)$ equations for the
determination of P, f, g_i, C_i, $i = 1-n$. Neglecting the $G(g_i)$
term in eqn. (29) in order to obtain the dominant approximation
g_{io} , C_{io} , it follows that

$$g_{io} = \{a_i(z)/[2/R - 2a_i(z)\ln R]\}(C_{io} - c_{i\infty}) , \quad (30)$$

and that

$$\frac{d}{dz}[C_{io} \frac{dP}{dz}] = a_i^*(z)[C_{io} - c_{i\infty}] \quad (31)$$

where $a_i^*(z) = a_i(z)/\gamma[1 - a_i(z)R \ln R]$. With the initial conditions $C_i(0) = 1$, $P'(0) = -Q_o$, the solution to eqn. (31) is

$$C_{io} = -\frac{1}{P'(z)} e^{\int_o^z \frac{a_i^*(\zeta)}{P'(\zeta)}d\zeta} \left\{ \hat{Q}_o + c_{i\infty} \int_o^z a_i^*(\zeta) e^{-\int_o^\zeta \frac{a_i^*(\eta)d\eta}{P'(\eta)}} d\zeta \right\}. \quad (32)$$

Assuming for the moment that $P(z)$ is a known function, eqn. (32)
gives the solution for $C_{io}(z)$, and eqn. (30) gives the solution
for $g_{io}(z)$. This solution for g_{io} can be used to evaluate
the neglected term $G(g_i)$ in eqn. (29) and an improved solution
g_{i1}, C_{i1}, obtained from the equations

$$\frac{2}{R} g_{i1} = a_i(z)[C_{i1}(z) - c_{i\infty} + 2g_{i1} \ln R - G(g_{io})] = \gamma \frac{d}{dz}[C_{i1} \frac{dP}{dz}] .$$

In a manner analogous to that used in obtaining the solution,
eqns. (30) and (32), it follows that

$$g_{i1} = (\gamma R/2)a_i^*(z)[C_{i1} - c_{i\infty} - G(g_{io})] \quad (33)$$

and

$$C_{io} = -\frac{1}{P'(z)} e^{\int_o^z \frac{a_i^*(\zeta)}{P'(\zeta)}d\zeta} \left\{ \hat{Q}_o + \int_o^z [c_{i\infty} + G(g_{io})]a_i^*(\zeta) e^{-\int_o^\zeta \frac{a_i^*(\eta)d\eta}{P'(\eta)}} d\zeta \right\}.$$

$$(34)$$

This procedure provides the basis for an iteration scheme, since
the new solution, $g_{i1}(z)$, can be substituted into the $G(g_i)$

term in eqn. (29) and the procedure repeated to find C_{i2}, g_{i2}. The iteration can be continued until convergence to any desired degree of accuracy is attained.

Having obtained the solution C_i, g_i for each of the species, $f(z)$ can be found from eqn. (28). Letting $\Psi(z) = \sum_{i=1}^{n} \beta_i \sigma_i(z)$ $[c_\infty - 2g_i \ell n \ R + G(g_i) - C_i(z)]$, which is a known function of z, the dominant solution for $f(z)$, denoted $f_0(z)$, is found by neglecting $G(f)$ in eqn. (28). Therefore $f_0(z) = K(z)\{P(z) - P_\infty + \Psi(z)\}/\{2/R - 2K(z)\ell n \ R\}$. An improved solution, $f_1(z)$, can be obtained by using $f_0(z)$ to evaluate the neglected term, $G(f)$. This gives $f_1(z) = K(z)\{P(z) - p_\infty + G(f_0) + \Psi(z)\}/\{2/R - 2K(z)\ell n \ R\}$. Again, an iteration scheme can be used to obtain a better solution, f_2, by using f_1 to evaluate $G(f)$. The procedure can be repeated until any desired degree of accuracy is attained.

The above solutions have been obtained by assuming that $P(z)$ is a known function. Since this is not the case, $P(z)$ will be assumed to be given by $1 - \hat{Q}_0 z$, an approximation that neglects the effect of fluid exchange on capillary pressure. Therefore, $P'(z) = -\hat{Q}_0$, and eqn. (32), for example, reduces to

$$C_{io} = c_{i\infty} + (1-c_{i\infty})\exp\{-(1/\hat{Q}_0) \int_0^z a_i^*(\zeta)d\zeta\} \ .$$

The entire procedure described above can therefore be carried out using this approximation for $P(z)$, and the solutions f, g_i, C_i obtained. Once this is completed, a better approximation for P can be obtained from eqn. (28), i.e., $d^2P/dZ^2 = (2/AR)f(z)$. Using the initial conditions $P(0) = 1$, $P'(0) = -\hat{Q}_0$, it follows that

$$P(z) = 1 - \hat{Q}_0 z + \frac{2}{AR}\left\{z \int_0^1 f(\nu)d\nu - \int_0^1 \nu f(\nu)d\nu\right\} \ . \tag{35}$$

This improved solution for $P(z)$ can then be used in the above scheme to obtain new solutions f, g_i and C_i. The procedure can be continually repeated to attain any desired degree of accuracy.

The analysis presented here has been used to study the effect of various mutually interacting metabolites on capillary-tissue exchange (Salathé and Venkataraman, in preparation). In all cases the iterative scheme described converged very rapidly and highly accurate solutions were obtained. It was found that a single metabolite delivered by blood to tissue, such as glucose, can exert sufficient osmotic pressure so that reabsorption occurs along the entire capillary length. Conversely, only filtration occurred if the osmotic effect was included for a single metabolite produced in the tissue, such as lactate. When both metabolites were included, however, a balance was achieved, with filtration at the arterial end and reabsorption at the venous end taking place.

When saturation in the capillary-tissue transport of the various metabolites occurs, the solution presented here is no longer valid. With saturation, when the concentration difference across the capillary wall for any metabolite exceeds a given level, no further transcapillary transport of this metabolite takes place. The analysis in this case is complicated by the fact that the capillary and tissue concentrations depend on the position along the capillary where saturation occurs, but this position is not known in advance and must be determined as part of the solution. Using techniques similar to those described in this section, such problems have been solved (Venkataraman and Salathé, in preparation) for any number of metabolites, under the general condition that the concentration difference at which saturation occurs and the amount of solute transported at saturation is a function of position along the capillary for each metabolite.

UNSTEADY PERIODIC PROBLEMS

Oscillations in capillary pressure resulting from periodic contractions of precapillary sphincters or feeding arterioles induce disturbances to the interstitial pressure and protein concentrations that are governed by eqns. (1) and (2). These fluctuations in capillary pressure cause fluid to be alternately filtered and reabsorbed from the capillary. When filtration occurs, interstitial fluid pressure increases from its background value as the capillary is approached, whereas for reabsorption the pressure decreases as the capillary is approached. If the oscillations are sufficiently slow, or if the tissue is sufficiently stiff ($\partial\theta/\partial p$ small), the unsteady term in eqn. (1) will be small and the governing equation for interstitial fluid pressure reduces to the steady form, $\nabla \cdot \theta K_+ \nabla p = 0$. For such cases the behavior is quasi-static, and as the capillary pressure varies the interstitial fluid pressure will pass through a sequence of profiles given by the steady solution. According to the steady theory, the oscillations in interstitial fluid pressure should persist for a distance from the capillary of several hundred microns. Wiederhielm and Weston [13] measured interstitial fluid pressure adjacent to capillaries in the web of the bat wing, and did not observe such fluctuations. This apparent paradox was resolved [8] by showing that the interstitial fluid pressure is in fact governed by the full unsteady form of eqn. (1), and that its behavior is very different from that described by the corresponding quasi-steady results. It was found that precapillary sphincter or arteriole contractions are high frequency oscillations, and the disturbances to interstitial fluid pressure created in the tissue decay in a few microns from the capillary. These conclusions were subsequently extended to the disturbances in extra-vascular protein concentrations [11].

If the changes in tissue porosity resulting from interstitial fluid pressure oscillations are sufficiently small, the expansion $\theta(p) \sim \theta(p_\infty) + \theta'(p_\infty)(p-p_\infty)$ holds and eqn. (1) can be linearized.

Henceforth in this section protein concentration will again be normalized by its value at the arterial end, all pressures will be normalized by the mean arterial pressure $\bar{P}_A$, distances will be normalized by capillary length L , and time by the half period of oscillation T . The linearized form of eqn. (1) is then

$$\frac{\partial p}{\partial t} - k_1 \nabla^2 p = 0 \qquad (36)$$

where $k_1 = \hat{\theta}_\infty \hat{K}_{t\infty} T / \hat{\theta}'_\infty L^2$.

Regarding the interstitial protein concentration as a small perturbation to its uniform value far from the capillary, eqn. (2) can be reduced to the linearized form

$$\frac{\partial c}{\partial t} - k_2 \nabla^2 c = 0 \qquad (37)$$

for the normalized concentration, where $k_2 = \hat{D}_\infty T / L^2$. Equation (36) and the assumption $\lambda = 1$ were used in obtaining this result.

If capillary protein leakage is neglected, the disturbances to interstitial protein concentration, as well as to interstitial fluid pressure, are a consequence only of capillary-tissue fluid exchange. This exchange is governed by Starling's law, eqn. (3). Consistent with the linearization, in this equation tissue hydrostatic and osmotic pressures can be replaced by their uniform values far from the capillary, the plasma osmotic pressure can be assumed constant, and the capillary pressure can be assumed to drop linearly from the arterial to the venous end. It then follows from eqns. (3) and (8) that p and c satisfy the following boundary conditions at the capillary wall:

$$\left.\frac{\partial p}{\partial r}\right|_R = -\frac{1}{\alpha}\left.\frac{\partial c}{\partial r}\right|_R = -K\{P_A(t) - [P_A(t) - P_v(t)]z - p_\infty + \pi_\infty - \Pi_0\} \qquad (38)$$

where $K = k_f L / \hat{\theta}_\infty \hat{K}_{t\infty}$, $\alpha = \hat{K}_{t\infty} \bar{P}_A c_\infty / \hat{D}_\infty$ are non-dimensional parameters, and $P_A(t)$, $P_v(t)$ are the normalized arterial and venous pressures. Equations (36) and (37) must be solved subject to the boundary conditions eqn. (38) and the condition that $p \to p_\infty$, $c \to c_\infty$ far from the capillary.

Since the equations and boundary conditions are linear, the pressure and concentration can be separated into a steady and unsteady part, $p = p_s + p_{us}$, $c = c_s + c_{us}$. The steady part satisfies the equation $\nabla^2 p_s = 0$, $\nabla^2 c_s = 0$, and predicts disturbances that decay over a distance from the capillary of the order of the capillary length. Since the steady problem was discussed in the previous two sections, it will not be considered further here.

For the unsteady part of the solution, it is appropriate to normalize radial distance with respect to the capillary radius R_c , while axial distance should remain normalized with respect to capillary length L . Denoting the renormalized radial distance by r^* , eqn. (26) becomes

$$\frac{\partial p}{\partial t} = -\frac{k_1 L^2}{R_c^2} \left\{ \frac{\partial^2 p}{\partial r^{*2}} + \frac{1}{r} \frac{\partial p}{\partial r^*} + \left(\frac{R_c}{L}\right)^2 \frac{\partial^2 p}{\partial z^2} \right\} . \tag{39}$$

In order to determine the constant k_1 it is necessary to specify the function $\theta(p)$. Using the experimental results of Guyton [3], it was found [8] that $k_1 L^2 / R_c^2$ is of the order of one. Therefore, the unsteady term and the radial derivatives are of the same order of magnitude, and since $(R_c/L)^2 << 1$ the unsteady disturbances to interstitial fluid pressure are governed by the equation

$$\frac{\partial p}{\partial t} + k_1 \left(\frac{\partial^2 p}{\partial r^2} + \frac{1}{r} \frac{\partial p}{\partial r}\right) = 0 . \tag{40}$$

The interstitial protein concentration is governed by an analogous equation [11].

Equation (40) can be solved by an eigenfunction expansion in terms of Bessel function of complex argument [8]. The solutions predict oscillations of several millimeters of mercury in the interstitial fluid pressure at the capillary wall. However, these oscillations decay to insignificant magnitude within a distance of a few capillary radii from the wall. This rapid decay in pressure fluctuations is a direct consequence of the dependence of porosity θ on interstitial fluid pressure. Since the alternating periods of filtration and reabsorption occur at high frequency, the filtered fluid can be stored in a thin layer of tissue adjacent to the capillary during the brief period of filtration until it is reabsorbed into the capillary. The decay distance is characterized by the parameter $\hat{\theta}_\infty \hat{K}_{t\infty} T^2 / \pi R_c^2 \hat{\theta}_\infty'$. Therefore, the ability of the tissue to store fluid in a thin collar requires a short period $(T<<1)$, large resistance to fluid movement $(\hat{\theta}_\infty \hat{K}_{t\infty} << 1)$, a highly compliant tissue $(\hat{\theta}_\infty' >> 1)$, and a large area of tissue available near the capillary $(\pi R_c^2 >> 1)$.

CONCLUSION

A very general single capillary model of capillary-tissue fluid exchange has been presented. Although the governing equations are extremely complex, considerable progress has been made in the development of appropriate mathematical methods for their solution. An extension of the non-linear solution discussed in Section 4 to include protein leakage by mechanisms other than solvent drag is needed. Also, there is a lack of experimental data from which to determine many of the functions appearing in the theory. Considerable activity is presently being devoted to determining $k_f(z)$, but little is known about the hydrodynamic conductivity and its dependence on interstitial fluid pressure and nothing is known about $D(p)$ and $\lambda(p)$. The analysis of the osmotic effect of numerous metabolites assumes that all these functions are constant, so that a linear theory results. It was assumed that the solutes do not interact in their passage across the capillary membrane. A coupling of their transport mechanisms can lead to much larger fluxes as well as movement of a solute against its own concentration gradient. The analysis of such facilitated diffusion, as well as various forms of active transport, would be an important extension of the present model.

The governing equations for interstitial fluid pressure and protein concentration were linearized in order to analyze unsteady phenomena. Consistent with the linearization, it was assumed that the dominant approximation to fluid movement is given by a simplified form of Starling's law in which the effect of filtration and reabsorption on the four Starling pressures can be neglected. While these simplifications are justified for a wide variety of physiological situations, there are important cases for which they are not valid. The development of a nonlinear unsteady solution would be a difficult but important undertaking.

The analysis of transient effects, such as the microcirculatory response following an occlusion, is generally more difficult than the analysis of periodic phenomena. One transient problem, the accumulation and eventual washout of osmotically active metabolites suddenly produced in a tissue, has recently been studied (Wang and Salathé, in preparation). It was found that such metabolites remain at high concentration and exert appreciable osmotic pressure in the tissue for several minutes after their production. This is in agreement with the theory that the rapid outpouring of fluid from capillaries immediately following burn injury is a result of osmotically active particles released in the tissue.

The analysis presented in this chapter is based strictly on a single capillary model. It is not applicable, for example, to skeletal muscle, which consists of a large number of closely spaced parallel capillaries. Also, these capillaries are imbedded in large muscle fibers that run parallel to the vessels, so that the concept of interstitial fluid motion presented here is not applicable. The model would also require modification for organs such as mesentery that have a thickness of the order of the capillary diameter. Since the mesentery itself exchanges fluid with its surroundings, this would have a significant effect on capillary-tissue fluid exchange.

In conclusion, therefore, a great deal of analytic study on capillary exchange remains to be done, not only in the further development of solutions to the equations presented here, but also in the development of models appropriate to tissue for which the present theory is not applicable.

REFERENCES

1. An, K. N., and Salathé, E. P. (1976): A theory of interstitial fluid motion and its implications for capillary exchange. Microvasc. Res., 12:103-119.
2. An, K. N., and Salathé, E. P. (1976): The effect of variable capillary radius and filtration coefficients on fluid exchange.

Biorheology, 13:367-378.

3. Guyton, A. C. (1965): Interstitial fluid pressure. II. Pressure-volume curves of interstitial space. Circulation Res., 16:452-460.

4. Guyton, A. C., Scheel, K., and Murphree, D. (1966): Interstitial fluid pressure. III. Its effect on resistance to tissue fluid mobility. Circulation Res., 19:412-419.

5. Landis, E. M. (1927): Micro-injection studies of capillary permeability, I. Amer. J. Physiol., 81:124-142.

6. Landis, E. M., and Pappenheimer, J. R. (1963): Exchange of substances through the capillary walls. In: Handbook of Physiology Circulation, edited by W. F. Hamilton and P. Dow, pp. 961-1034. Waverly Press, New York.

7. McMaster, P. D. (1941): An inquiry into structural conditions effecting fluid transport in the interstitial tissue of the skin. J. Exptl. Med., 74:9-28.

8. Salathé, E. P. (1977): An analysis of interstitial fluid pressure in the web of the bat wing. Amer. J. Physiol., 232: H297-H304 or Amer. J. Physiol.: Heart Circ. Physiol., 1:H297-H304.

9. Salathé, E. P., and An, K. N. (1976): A mathematical analysis of fluid movement across capillary walls. Microvasc. Res., 11:1-23.

10. Salathé, E. P., and Venkataraman, R. (1978): Role of extravascular protein in capillary-tissue fluid exchange. Amer. J. Physiol., 234:H52-H58 or Amer. J. Physiol.: Heart Circ. Physiol., 3:H52-H58.

11. Salathé, E. P., Venkataraman, R., and Gross, J. F. (1979): Microcirculatory response to periodic pulsations in capillary pressure. (To appear)

12. Wiederhielm, C. A. (1972): The interstitial space. In: Biomechanics, Its Foundations and Objectives, edited by Y. C. Fung, N. Perrone, and M. Anliker, pp. 273-285. Prentice Hall, Englewood Cliffs, New Jersey.

13. Wiederhielm, C. A., and Weston, B. V. (1973): Microvascular, lymphatic, and tissue pressures in the unanesthetized mammal. Amer. J. Physiol., 225:992-996.

14. Yoffey, J. M., and Courtice, F. C. (1970): Lymphatics, Lymph and the Lymphomyeloid Complex. Academic Press, New York.

Mathematics of Microcirculation Phenomena,
edited by J. F. Gross and A. Popel.
Raven Press, New York © 1980.

Vesicular Transport of Macromolecules Across Vascular Endothelium

Sheldon Weinbaum and *Shu Chien

*Department of Mechanical Engineering, The City College of The City University of New York, New York, New York 10031, and *Division of Circulatory Physiology and Biophysics, Department of Physiology, Columbia University College of Physicians and Surgeons, New York, New York 10032*

INTRODUCTION

Physiological Background

The transport of proteins and other macromolecules across cell membranes is an important physiological process. The endothelial cells lining the vascular system regulate the passage of macromolecules such that protein concentrations in the interstitial space differ from those in the plasma. The maintenance of a protein concentration gradient across the capillary endothelium serves to provide the difference in colloidal osmotic pressure governing transcapillary fluid transfer (9). The controlled transfer of proteins and lipoproteins between plasma and arterial wall through the arterial endothelium plays a significant role in regulating the metabolism and maintaining homeostasis in the arterial wall (4). Therefore, an understanding of the mechanisms governing protein transport across vascular endothelium can help to elucidate several basic physiological processes in the vascular system and to provide insights into the pathophysiological basis of such disease states as edema and atherosclerosis.

Since the initial investigations by Palade (11), there is increasing evidence that transendothelial transport of macromolecules, especially those larger than 40 Å in diameter, is mediated primarily by the plasmalemmal vesicles. These endothelial vesicles can be seen on electron micrographs of thin

sections or replicas of freeze fracture preparations of blood
vessels (Fig. 1). With the use of transmission electron micro-
scopy, electron dense markers larger than 40 Å are seen to traverse the endothelial cells via the vesicles rather than the
intercellular clefts (17). The results of physiological investigations with the use of tracers with various molecular sizes
are in general agreement with the concept that macromolecules
larger than 40 Å pass through the capillary endothelium via a
"large pore" system, which is most likely the vesicles (13).

The mechanisms of vesicle attachment and detachment have
been postulated on the basis of electron microscopic findings

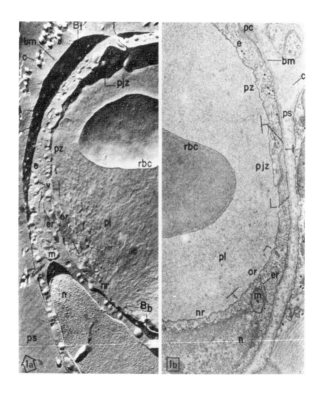

FIG. 1. Comparison between a replica of a nearly transverse fracture through a blood capillary of rat diaphragm (1a,
x22,600) and a section (1b, x20,600). The fracture exposes the
B face of the plasmalemma on the tissue front at B_t and the A
and B faces of the plasmalemma on the blood front at A_b and
B_b, respectively. From Simionescu et al. (18).

(12) on the shape of vesicles near the plasmalemma (Fig. 2).
When the vesicle arrives at the vicinty of the plasmalemma, molecular interaction forces between the opposing membranes cause
their deformation and contact, eventually leading to membrane
breakdown in the middle of the contact area and membrane fusion
in the rim. Vesicle detachment may be the result of large
amplitude deformation at the stalk due to the collective behavior of many thermal collisions with water molecules (1, 2),
leading to wave propagation in the stalk and its rupture. There
have been several investigations on the dynamic behavior of
vesicle transport by the use of electron dense markers in time
dependent studies (3, 17). In their quantitative studies on
the mouse heart capillary endothelium and diaphragm mesothelium,
Casley-Smith and Chin (3) determined the proportion of cyto-
plasmic vesicles containing markers (ferritin, horseradish
peroxidase and sodium ferrocyanide) as a function of the distance through the cell at various time intervals after tracer
introduction. They showed that the concentration profile of
the labeled vesicles grew with time, reaching a steady state in
approximately 10 sec.

The ultrastructural and functional information available on
arterial transport has provided the impetus for the present theoretical modeling of vesicle dynamics, with the aim of elucidating the fundamental mechanism of transendothelial transport of
macromolecules.

Theoretical Models

In the past decade a variety of theoretical models have
been introduced to quantitatively analyze both the steady state
vesicle transport process (8, 15, 16, 19, 20) and the time
dependent labeling experiments (1, 2, 14) described in the
physiological introduction. The earliest of the steady state

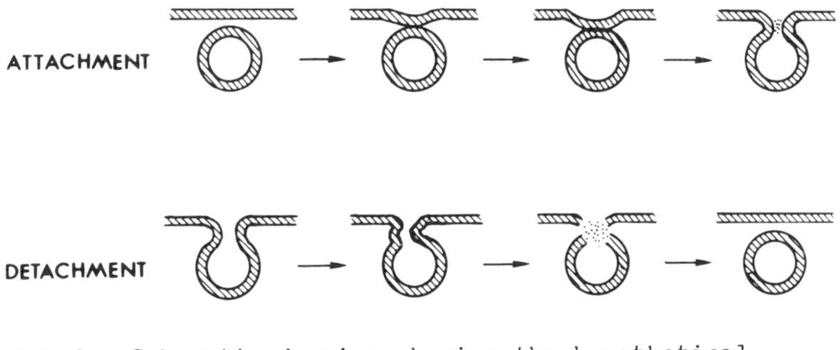

FIG. 2. Schematic drawing showing the hypothetical
processes of attachment of the endtothelial vesicle to the
plasmalemmal membrane (stages shown in upper drawings) and the
detachment of the vesicle from the membrane (stages shown in
lower drawings).

models were based on one-dimensional continuum diffusion theory
(19) or random walk computer simulation experiments (16) in
which the interaction of the vesicle with the boundary plasmalemmal membranes was neglected entirely and a constant diffusion
coefficient assumed based on infinite domain Stokes-Einstein
diffusion theory. Because of the poor agreement of the predicted steady state concentration profiles and the available
experimental data, it was soon realized that events near the
plasmalemma played a vital role in the transport process. To
remedy this shortcoming, Green and Casley-Smith (8) and Shea
and Bossert (15) propose an ad hoc phenomenological approach in
which the wall is modeled as an imperfectly absorbing barrier
with an elastic reflection coefficient α. The value of α is
empirically determined so as to provide a reasonable curve fit
with the experimental data.

The first dynamic model of the steady state vesicle transport process, which attempts to consider in an approximate
manner the hydrodynamic and molecular force interactions between
the vesicle and the plasmalemma, is presented in Weinbaum and
Caro (1976). In this model, whose key features are summarized
in the next section, a theoretical expression is derived for the
spatial variation of the diffusion coefficient, which takes into
account the increased hydrodynamic resistance of the vesicle as
it approaches the plasmalemmal membranes on each side of the
cell, and for the van der Waals electrodynamic attractive force
between the vesicle and the boundary plasmalemmal membranes.
This more complete model still neglects (a) the chemical and
elastic deformation energies involved in the formation and dissolution of vesicle attachment stalks, (b) the steric hindrance
due to the crowding of attached vesicles, (c) collisions between
vesicles, and (d) electric double layer forces. The first two
factors are now known to play an important role in the overall
vesicle dynamics, whereas the third and fourth factors are believed to be less significant since the average spacing between
free vesicles is several diameters (12) and the negative surface
charge on plasmalemmal membranes is normally found on their
exterior rather than their interior faces (10).

The first of the above factors, the formation and dissolution of the vesicle stalk, is treated as a free energy barrier
within the framework of absolute reaction rate theory in Rubin
(14). This last paper also shows how the processes of vesicle
attachment/detachment can be related to the diffusion of the
free vesicles in the cell interior to define a steady state permeability coefficient for the entire vesicle transport process.
The second factor, the steric hindrance of closely spaced attached vesicles, was clearly demonstrated by Simionescu et al.
(17) using the freeze cleavage technique, but omitted from the
theoretical modeling because there was no theory available to
describe how the spatial variation of the vesicle diffusion coefficient would be modified by the vesicle attachment density.
At the time of this writing, laboratory model experiments for

predicting this steric exclusion effect have been combined with the recent, more accurate solutions of Ganatos et al. (7) for the transverse creeping motion of a sphere between parallel planar walls to provide much more realistic expressions for the vesicle diffusion coefficient in the cell interior than previously available. The first results of this work, which will be reported on in greater detail later this year (2), show very encouraging agreement with the steady state vesicle concentration profiles observed by Casley-Smith and Chin (3).

Rubin (14) also presents a simplified time dependent theoretical model which provides rough qualitative agreement with the initial stages of time dependent vesicle labeling experiments. The vesicle motion in the cell interior is described by a one-dimensional, unsteady diffusion with a constant diffusion coefficient, while the process of vesicle attachment/detachment at the luminal surface is described by the same reaction rate theory used in the steady state models. Solutions are presented for the case where the abluminal plasmalemmal membrane is assumed to be at infinity and the processes of vesicle attachment/detachment are considered to be a mirror image sequence of events. These solutions are valid for only very early times, because of the neglect of the second plasmalemmal membrane, and can not be used to describe the approach to steady state labeling. It is also clear from the ultrastructural studies described in the introduction that the processes of vesicle attachment/detachment probably are not symmetric (Fig. 2). The time that a vesicle resides in its open attached state before vesicle stalk dissolution is much longer than the process of vesicle stalk formation once initial contact between the vesicle and the plasmalemma has occurred. Also, the sequence of membrane shapes is not reversible. The more recent time dependent theory of Arminski et al. (1) combines the reaction rate theory approach of Rubin (14), modified to take account of the asymmetry of the vesicle attachment/detachment processes just described, with the spatially nonuniform diffusion theory of Weinbaum and Caro (20) extended to unsteady one-dimensional diffusion. This theory, which considers both boundary plasmalemmal membranes and the effect of near field electrodynamic forces, is described in some detail in the section on Mathematical Formulation.

In addition to the steady and unsteady vesicle models summarized in this section, we have also proposed a quantitative model (to be published) to describe the enhancement of vesicle transport produced by mechanical stretch and pressure oscillations of vessel length. This model assumes that the mechanical deformation of the endothelial cells creates irreversible intracellular currents which reduce transendothelial vesicle diffusion time but do not alter vesicle attachment time, since the boundary velocities created by disturbances with frequencies in the physiological range are small compared to the thermally induced deformation velocities of the vesicle.

MATHEMATICAL FORMULATION

The theoretical models summarized in the last section are conveniently divided into four categories: (a) steady state diffusion, (b) steady state permeability, (c) time dependent vesicle labeling and (d) mechanically enhanced transport. The key assumptions that are common to all the models described in this survey are:

(i) the vesicle transport process is passive and except for the process of vesicle stalk formation derives its energy from thermal motions,

(ii) the process is one-dimensional with equal numbers of vesicles being released at the luminal and abluminal surfaces, and

(iii) the total vesicle population (free plus attached) is constant.

Steady State Diffusion

In this category we shall consider in detail only the spatially varying diffusivity model of Weinbaum and Caro (20), since this model reduces to the earlier constant diffusivity theories (14, 15, 16, 19) if the hydrodynamic and van der Waals force interactions between the vesicle and the plasmalemmal membranes are neglected. Also, the mechanism of a fluid resistance barrier for squeezing out the water film between the vesicle and the plasmalemma is equivalent to having an imperfectly absorbing barrier (8, 15) in the constant diffusivity models.

Fig. 3 is a schematic illustration showing the simplified geometry and typical dimensions for the diffusion of a vesicle across an endothelial cell. As shown in this sketch the

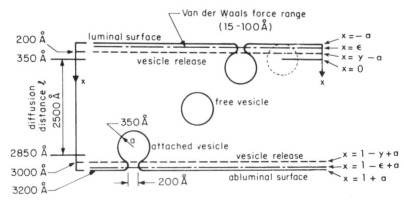

FIG. 3. Sketch of mathematical model showing typical dimensions for the transendothelial motion of a vesicle between parallel plasmalemmas.

vesicles are assumed to be symmetrically released from each
plasmalemma at a finite distance $y = 200$ Å, which is equal to
the length of the vesicle attachment stalk. The distance
between the plasmalemmas is equal to the diffusion distance of
the center of vesicle ℓ plus the vesicle diameter 2a representing the excluded distance of the vesicle center from the two
boundary membranes. In the vicinity of each plasmalemma it is
hypothesized that there exist narrow regions ε with typical
dimensions of from 15 to 100 Å where electrodynamic attractive
forces are important. The origin of coordinate $x = 0$ is
measured from the center of the vesicle if the vesicle surface
were to touch the luminal surface.

Since the process is symmetric for the two plasmalemmas we
need consider only vesicles released at the luminal side. The
governing steady state diffusion equation proposed which considers both the hydrodynamic and electrodynamic interactions
between the vesicle and the boundary membranes is

$$\frac{d(cu_{vw})}{dx} = \frac{d}{dx}\left(D(x)\frac{dc}{dx}\right) \qquad \begin{array}{c} 0 \leq x < y \\ y < x \leq 1 \end{array} \qquad (1)$$

where u_{vw} is a convective velocity imposed by the van der
Waals forces and $D(x)$ is a spatially dependent diffusion coefficient that describes the fluid resistance for a spherical
particle moving perpendicular to two plane parallel boundaries.
All distances in equation (1) and subsequently shall be scaled
relative to the diffusion distance ℓ. At the plane of release
$x = y$ we require that the solution to equation (1) in each
region satisfy

$$c(y^-) = c(y^+) \qquad (2)$$

$$\phi = D(y)\left(\frac{dc(y^-)}{dx} - \frac{dc(y^+)}{dx}\right) \qquad (3)$$

where ϕ is the vesicle release rate per unit area of luminal
surface.

The expression for u_{vw} is obtained by taking a force
balance on the vesicle in which the sum of van der Waals,
concentration gradient and hydrodynamic resistance forces is
set equal to zero.

$$0 = F_{vw} + 6\pi a\mu\lambda u_D - 6\pi a\mu\lambda u \qquad (4)$$

Here λ is a spatially varying hydrodynamic resistance coefficient which will be described shortly, and the total velocity u
is the sum of the Brownian diffusion velocity u_D and u_{vw}.
An approximate expression for the macroscopic force of attraction F_{vw} between the vesicle and the adjacent plasmalemma can

be obtained by integrating the non-retarded binary interaction
potential between all surface elements, neglecting all inter-
ference effects. This resultant force is

$$F_{vw} = \frac{3}{2} \pi^2 k \left(\frac{1}{x^4} - \frac{1}{(x+a)^4} \right) \qquad (5)$$

where k is proportional to the surface density of molecules and
the difference in the polarization properties of the bilayer
membrane and the intervening fluid.
    The derivation of an accurate expression for λ, even when
the steric hindrance of attached vesicles is neglected, is a
formidable mathematical problem. Exact solutions to the creeping motion equations for the transverse motion of a sphere
between infinite parallel boundaries have recently been obtained
by Ganatos et al. (7). In Weinbaum and Caro (20) a simple ad
hoc approximate expression is introduced

$$\lambda = 1 + \frac{a}{x} + \frac{a}{1-x} \qquad (6)$$

which approaches the correct limiting behavior as the fluid gap
shrinks to zero at each plasmalemmal membrane. Also, for x >> a
and λ = 1, one retrieves the well known Stokes formula for the
drag on an isolated sphere. Substituting results (5) and (6)
in equation (4) and defining x = ϵ_0 as the distance from the
luminal plasmalemma where u = $2u_D$ ($u_{vw} = u_D$), one can show
after some algebra

$$\frac{u}{u_D} = 1 + \left(\frac{\epsilon_0}{x}\right)^3 \left(\frac{1 + \frac{a}{\epsilon_0}}{\frac{x}{\epsilon_0} + \frac{a}{\epsilon_0}} \right)^5 \frac{(\frac{a}{\epsilon_0} + \frac{x}{\epsilon_0})^4 - (\frac{x}{\epsilon_0})^4}{(\frac{a}{\epsilon_0} + 1)^4 - 1} \qquad (7)$$

Fig. 4 is a plot based on equation (7) showing how the vesicle
velocity dramatically increases as the plasmalemma is approached. An important simplifying feature evident from Fig. 4
is that when a/ϵ_0 > 3.5 the solution for u is nearly independent of this parameter and equation (7) can be approximated by
the much simpler result

$$\frac{u}{u_D} \simeq 1 + \left(\frac{\epsilon_0}{x}\right)^3 \qquad (8)$$

    Equation (1) is first solved in the region close to the
luminal plasmalemma by neglecting the influence of the distant
boundary, i.e. the third term in equation (6) for λ, and using
approximation (8). In general, the spatial variation of the
vesicle diffusion coefficient is related to λ by

$$D(x) = D_O \lambda(x) \tag{9}$$

where D_O is the diffusion coefficient for a spherical particle in an infinite medium. The above near field solution for c which satisfies the condition that the free vesicle concentration vanishes at x = 0 is

$$c = \frac{aA}{3D_O} \ln\left(1 + \left(\frac{x}{\varepsilon_O}\right)^3\right) \tag{10}$$

where A is an unknown constant to be determined shortly by matching with the solution for c in the cell interior.

Fig. 5 is a plot of equation (10) showing the significant depletion of free vesicles near the plasmalemma that occurs due to the van der Waals attractive forces. Also shown in this figure (dashed curve) is the solution if the van der Waals forces are neglected. One notes that for this dashed curve c would appear to vanish at some fictitious location x = ε inside the cell. This distance, which we define as the effective van der Waals displacement distance, turns out to be exactly equal to ε_O when approximation (8) is used.

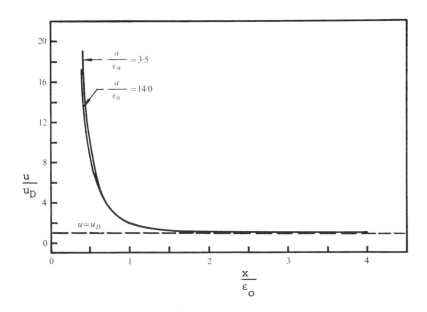

FIG. 4. Plot of equation (7) showing how the total vesicle velocity u is increased by van der Waals attraction near the plasmalemma. From Weinbaum and Caro (20).

Equation (1) is greatly simplified when one moves away from the thin layers of $O(\varepsilon)$ near each plasmalemma. In this interior region, $u_{VW} = 0$ and the effect of the van der Waals forces can be approximated by simply relocating the position at which the free vesicle concentration vanishes in accord with the above definition of the van der Waals displacement distance. Thus, we require for the interior solution that

$$c = 0 \qquad \text{at } x = \varepsilon \qquad\qquad (11)$$
$$c = 0 \qquad \text{at } x = 1 - \varepsilon \qquad\qquad (12)$$

The solution to equation (1) in the cell interior can be generalized to an arbitrary one-dimensional spatial distribution for $\lambda(x)$ and hence $D(x)$ by noting that the transformation

$$d\zeta = \lambda(x)\,dx \qquad\qquad (13)$$

reduces equation (1), when $u_{VW} = 0$, to the constant coefficient equation

$$\frac{d^2 c}{d\zeta^2} = 0 \qquad\qquad \begin{array}{l} \varepsilon \le x < y \\ y > x \ge 1 - \varepsilon \end{array} \qquad\qquad (14)$$

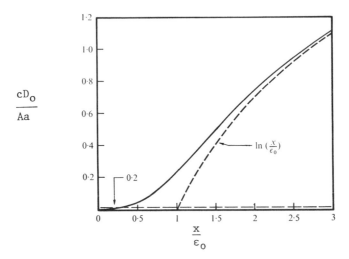

FIG. 5. Solid curve, plot of equation (10) for the dimensionless free vesicle concentration cD_0/aA. Dashed curve, solution if van der Waals forces are absent. From Weinbaum and Caro (20).

Similarly, matching condition (3) simplifies to

$$\frac{\ell\phi}{D_o} = \frac{dc(y^-)}{d\zeta} - \frac{dc(y^+)}{d\zeta} \tag{15}$$

Subjecting the integrating equation (14) to boundary and matching conditions (2), (11), (12) and (15), one obtains for an arbitrary distribution for $\lambda(x)$

$$c(x) = \frac{\ell\phi}{D_o}\left(1 - \frac{\zeta(y)}{\zeta(1-y)}\right)\zeta(x) \qquad \epsilon \leq x < y \tag{16a}$$

$$c(x) = \frac{\ell\phi}{D_o}\left(1 - \frac{\zeta(x)}{\zeta(1-\epsilon)}\right)\zeta(y) \qquad y < x \leq 1-\epsilon \tag{16b}$$

When λ is given by equation (6), equation (3) is readily integrated to yield

$$\zeta(x) = x - \epsilon + a\,\ln\frac{x(1-\epsilon)}{(1-x)\epsilon} \tag{17}$$

where the origin $\zeta = 0$ is chosen for convenience to be at $x = \epsilon$.

The solutions (16) for free vesicle concentration in the cell interior based on the hydrodynamic resistance distribution (equation 6) are plotted in Fig. 6 for several representative

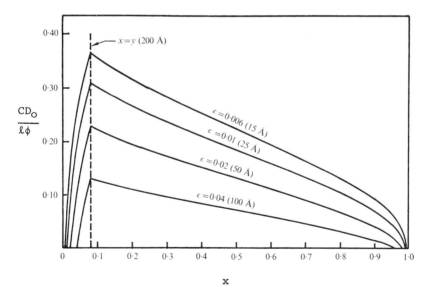

FIG. 6. Plot based on equations (16) and (17) of the dimensionless free vesicle concentration $CD_o/\ell\phi$ as a function of the dimensionless diffusion distance from the luminal for representative values of ϵ, $\ell = 2500$ Å. From Weinbaum and Caro (20).

values of ε. Since the van der Waals displacement thickness is small compared to the total transendothelial diffusion distance, one might expect the concentration profiles to be insensitive to changes in ε. As shown in Fig. 6 this is not the case. Because of the large increase in hydrodynamic resistance as the fluid gap narrows to distances less than the vesicle radius, the probability that a vesicle released at x = y will cross the cell rather than reattaching at the same plasmalemma from which it was released increases rapidly as the distance between x = ε and x = y, and hence the fluid resistance for reattachment, increases. This increase in the probability for transendothelial vesicle diffusion is manifested in Fig. 6 as a substantial increase in the total population of free vesicles (area under the concentration profile curves shown in Fig. 6).

The c profiles given by equations (10) and (16) can be asymptotically matched for large values of x/ε_0. The value of the constant A determined in this manner is

$$A = \ell\phi \left(1 - \frac{\zeta(y)}{\zeta(1-y)} \right) \tag{18}$$

The overlapping validity of solutions (10) and (16) near x = 0 is difficult to draw on the length scale of Fig. 6, but is easily seen on the scale of the expanded near field coordinate shown in Fig. 5. Note also that all the curves near the left hand side of Fig. 6 reduce to a single curve when the near field scaling shown in Fig. 5 is used.

Steady State Permeability

Rubin (14) has shown how the kinetics of the vesicle attachment/detachment process can be coupled to the diffusion in the cell interior and a steady state permeability coefficient defined for the overall vesicle transport process across the endothelial cell layer. The steady state permeability coefficient P is defined by

$$P = \frac{J}{C_p - C(o)} \tag{19}$$

where C_p and $C(o)$ are the macromolecule concentrations at the luminal and tissue surfaces of the endothelial cell, and J = $\phi_R V(C_p - C(o))$ is the net macromolecule flux from the lumen to the tissue front. ϕ_R is the vesicle number flux/cm^2 that crosses the cell, and V is the available filling volume in the vesicle interior. The preceding expression for J assumes that the vesicle attachment time t_a is long compared to the time that it takes the macromolecules to achieve concentration equilibrium with the luminal fluid. Experiments with large tracer molecules, such as ferritin (3, 6), strongly suggests that molecular sieving effects for these molecules may play an

important role in vesicle filling. This effect is easily
accounted for in the present analysis by multiplying the above
expression for J by an exponential factor $\exp(-t_f/t_a)$, which
describes a diffusion barrier with characteristic passage time
t_f at the mouth of the vesicle.

The probability in the steady state that a vesicle will
cross the cell once it is released ϕ_R/ϕ is readily obtained
from equation (16) by calculating the concentration gradients
on each side of the plane of release. This probability is
given by

$$\phi_R/\phi = \frac{\zeta(y)}{\zeta(1-\epsilon)} \qquad (20)$$

The vesicle release rate/cm^2 ϕ is related to the number
density/cm^2 of attached vesicles at the luminal surface N_a
by $\phi = N_a/t_a$. Combining equations (19), (20) and this
definition of ϕ, one obtains

$$P = \frac{N_a}{t_a} \left(\frac{\zeta(y)}{\zeta(1-y)} \right) V \qquad (21)$$

Using the notation introduced by Rubin (14), one writes
the total vesicle attachment time t_a as the sum of vesicle
stalk formation and dissolution times,

$$t_a = \frac{1}{k^d_1} + \frac{1}{k^d_{-1}} \qquad (22)$$

The rate constant k^d_{-1} describes the dissolution of the
vesicle and plasmalemmal membranes after contact and the formation of the vesicle stalk while the rate constant k^d_1
describes the rupture of the vesicle stalk and the resealing of
the vesicle membrane. The total vesicle density/cm^2 of endothelial surface is defined as $N = 2N_a + N_f$, where N_f is
the free vesicle density/cm^2. It is convenient to introduce
a dimensionless free vesicle density $N_f^* = (N_f D_o/\phi \ell^2)$.
N_f^* is readily found by integrating the concentration profiles (16 a,b) across the cell:

$$N_f^* = \int_0^{(1-\epsilon)} c d\zeta = \frac{1}{2}\left(\zeta(1-\epsilon)-\zeta(y)\right)\zeta(y) \qquad (23)$$

Substituting these results in equation (21), one obtains after
some algebra

$$P = \left(\frac{NVk^d_1}{2}\right)\left(\frac{\zeta(y)}{\zeta(1-\epsilon)}\right) \frac{1}{1 + \frac{k^d_1}{k^d_{-1}} + \frac{N_f^* \ell^2 k^d_1}{2D_o}} \qquad (24)$$

Equation (24) is valid for an arbitrary hydrodynamic resis-
tance distribution $\lambda(x)$. One simply specifies the function $\lambda(x)$
and intregrates equation (13) to obtain the function $\zeta(x)$ that
appears in equation (24) and the expression for N_f^* in equation (23). In Arminski et al. (1, 2) equation (6) is replaced
by the more general expression

$$\lambda = \beta + \frac{\theta a}{x} + \frac{\theta a}{1-x} \qquad (6a)$$

where the constants β and θ are selected to provide an optimum
root mean square curve fit with either the exact solutions of
Ganatos et al. (7) for the transverse motion of a sphere between infinite parallel boundaries or laboratory model experiments simulating the steric hindrance of attached vesicles.
  Equation 24 is plotted in Fig. 7 for $k^d_1/k^d_{-1} \ll 1$ and a λ
based on the exact solutions of Ganatos et al. (7). The parameter $\ell^2 k^d_1/2D_0$ is characteristic of vesicle diffusion to attachment times. The limits $\ell^2 k^d_1/2D_0 \gg 1$ and $\ell^2 k^d_1/2D_0 \ll 1$
thus represent the diffusion and attachment dominated limits
respectively. One observes that when $\ell^2 k^d_1/2D_0 \ll 1$ the permeability is controlled by the probability ϕ_R/ϕ that the vesicle
will cross the cell and thus is a sensitive function of ϵ.

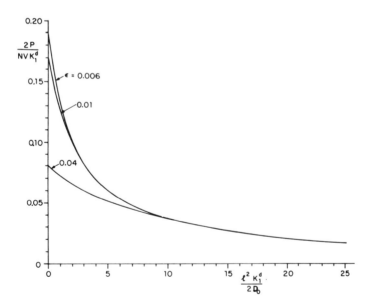

FIG. 7. Plot of the dimensionless permeability coefficient
$2P/NVk^d_1$ as a function of $\ell^2 k^d_1/2D_0$ for the same values
of ϵ and cell geometry as the curves in Fig. 6, based on equation (24), $k^d_1 \ll k^d_{-1}$. From Arminski et al. (1). λ based
on optimum curve fit to exact solution (7).

When $\ell^2 k^d{}_1/2D_0 \gg 1$ the increase in the free vesicle
density function N_f^* with decreasing ϵ just cancels the
increase in probability that the vesicle will cross the cell,
with the result that the steady state permeability is independent
of ϵ.

Time Dependent Vesicle Labeling

As described in the introduction, experiments to study
vesicular transport are usually conducted by introducing at
some time t = 0 a labeled marker molecule and then studying the
subsequent advance of the labeled vesicles at different time
intervals across the cell. This time dependent behavior has
been examined in Arminiski et al. (1) by including an unsteady
term in equation (1)

$$\frac{\partial c}{\partial t} + \frac{\partial (cu_{VW})}{\partial x} = \frac{\partial}{\partial x}\left(D(x)\frac{\partial c}{\partial x}\right) \qquad \begin{array}{l} 0 \le x < y \\ y < x \le 1 \end{array} \qquad (25a,b)$$

The boundary value problem for equations (25 a,b) is much
more difficult to solve than its steady state counterpart. Even
using the rather severe simplifying assumption of constant diffusivity one is unable to solve the unsteady problem by analytical methods if the effect of both plasmalemmal membranes is to be
included. Rubin (14) thus solves equation (25) for D constant,
treating the cell interior as infinite. One simplifying feature,
easily demonstrated by order of magnitude dimensional anaylsis,
is that the characteristic time required to achieve a quasi-
steady vesicle concentration profile in the thin van der Waals
force layers near each plasmalemma is of $O(\epsilon a/\ell^2)$ smaller than
the time required to achieve a steady state profile for the
entire cell. This implies that the labeled vesicles in the
regions $0 \le x \le \epsilon$ and $1-\epsilon \le x \le 1$ can be treated as though they
go through a sequence of quasi-steady states in which the concen-
tration is slowly changing on the time scale of the unsteady
diffusion in the cell interior. Equation (10), the solution for
the vesicle concentration profile in the electrodynamic layer
near the luminal membrane, still applies but the coefficient A is
no longer constant but a slowly varying function of time that is
obtained by matching with the unsteady solution in the cell
interior.

In the interior of the cell, outside the van der Waals
layers, equations (25) can be made dimensionless by introducing
the scaled variables $x^* = x/\ell$, $t^* = tD_0/\ell^2$ and $C^* = CD_0/\ell\phi$
and written in the more convenient form

$$\frac{\partial c^*}{\partial t^*} = \lambda(\zeta)\frac{\partial^2 c^*}{\partial \zeta^2} \qquad \begin{array}{l} \epsilon \le x < y \\ y < x \le 1-\epsilon \end{array} \qquad (26a,b)$$

after applying the coordinate transformation given in equation
(13). The boundary and matching conditions for equations
(26 a,b) are equations (11), (12), (2), and (3)or(15). Matching
conditions (2) and (3) are now, however, time dependent since
both c and its gradient are unknown functions of time that must
be determined as part of the solution. The initial condition
corresponding to most experiments is

$$c = 0 \qquad\qquad t \leq 0 \qquad\qquad (27)$$

The boundary value problem outlined in the last paragraph
cannot be solved in closed form, even if λ is a constant, because
of the complication introduced by the time dependent matching
conditions (2) and (3). To circumvent the considerable time and
expense that would be required in a numerical finite difference
solution scheme, Arminski et al. (1, 2) adopt an approximate
integral solution technique in which equations (26 a,b) are converted to first order ordinary differential equations. The con-
ceptual outline of the solution procedure is illustrated in
Fig. 8. We consider two concentration boundary layers of thicknesses $\delta_1(t)$ and $\delta_2(t)$ spreading with time from the vesicle
plane of release x = y. There are three different time domains
of solution. For $t \leq t_1$ both boundary layers grow until the
one on the left reaches x = ϵ and $\delta_1(t_1)$ = y-ϵ. The boundary layer to the right has not yet reached x = 1-ϵ.

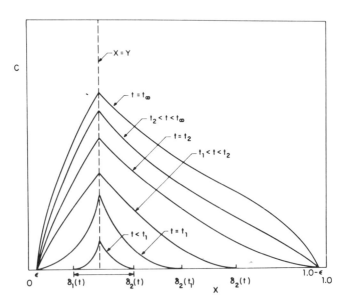

FIG. 8. Sketch showing three time domains for labeled
vesicle concentration profiles in intregral solution technique.
From Arminski et al. (1).

This marks the beginning of the second time domain $t_1 \leq t \leq t_2$. In this time domain the boundary layer on the right continues to grow towards $x = 1-\varepsilon$, while the one on the left remains fixed at $x = \varepsilon$, where it satisfies condition (11), but with a time dependent concentration gradient given by equation (28 a) below at $x = \varepsilon$. This behavior continues until the boundary layer on the right reaches $x = 1-\varepsilon$ and $\delta_2(t_2) = 1-\varepsilon-y$. In the third time domain $t_2 \leq t < t_{\infty}$, both boundary layers satisfy equations (11) or (12) at the effective edge of the van der Waals layers $x = \varepsilon$ and $x = 1-\varepsilon$, but their concentration gradients at these locations will vary until a steady state concentration profile is asymptotically achieved. The transformed concentration gradients at the edge of the boundary layers therefore satisfy the conditions

$$\frac{\partial c^*}{\partial \zeta} = 0 \qquad x = y-\delta_1 \qquad t^* < t_1^* \qquad (28a)$$

$$\frac{\partial c^*}{\partial \zeta} = \alpha_1(t^*) \qquad x = y-\varepsilon \qquad t^* > t_1^* \qquad (28b)$$

$$\frac{\partial c^*}{\partial \zeta} = 0 \qquad x = y+\delta_2 \qquad t^* < t_2^* \qquad (29a)$$

$$\frac{\partial c^*}{\partial \zeta} = \alpha_2(t^*) \qquad x = 1-y-\varepsilon \qquad t^* > t_2^* \qquad (29b)$$

where $\alpha_1(t^*)$ and $\alpha_2(t^*)$ are unknown functions of time. In summary, one must determine $\delta_1(t^*)$ and $\delta_2(t^*)$ for $0 \leq t^* \leq t_1^*$, $\alpha_1(t^*)$ and $\delta_2(t^*)$ for $t_1^* \leq t^* \leq t_2^*$, and $\alpha_1(t^*)$ and $\alpha_2(t^*)$ for $t^* > t_2^*$.

In the integral average technique equations (26 a,b) are replaced by the integral average equations

$$\int \frac{\partial c^*}{\partial t^*} d\zeta = \int \lambda(\zeta) \frac{\partial^2 c^*}{\partial \zeta^2} d\zeta \qquad \begin{array}{l} \zeta(\varepsilon) \leq \zeta < \zeta(y) \\ \zeta(y) < \zeta \leq \zeta(1-\varepsilon) \end{array} \qquad (30a,b)$$

and a suitable analytic form selected for the concentration profile in each boundary layer. One mathematically convenient set of profiles, which has the advantage that it reduces exactly to the solutions (16 a,b) in the steady state, is the polynomial description

$$c^* = a_1(t^*) + a_2(t^*)\zeta + a_3(t^*)\zeta^2 \qquad x < y \qquad (31a)$$

$$c^* = a_4(t^*) + a_5(t^*)\zeta + a_6(t^*)\zeta^2 \qquad x > y \qquad (31b)$$

The six unknown coefficents a_i, $i = 1, 2...6$, are first determined by satisfying boundary or matching conditions (2), (11), (12) and (15) applied at $x = y$ and the boundary layer edge and two appropriate conditions from (28) and (29). In this manner all the a_i can be expressed in terms of two unknown functions from the set δ_1, δ_2, α_1 and α_2 depending on the time domain of

interest. When profiles (31 a,b) are substituted in equations
(30 a,b) and the integrations performed, one obtains two coupled
first order ordinary differential equations for the boundary
layer thickness or the transformed concentration gradient at
its edge in each of the three time domains sketched in Fig. 8.

The ease with which the above solution procedure can be
carried to completion depends in large measure on the form of
the approximating function used to describe the spatial distribution $\lambda(x)$ of the hydrodynamic resistance. One would like to
be able to integrate equation (13) in closed form, analytically
evaluate the integrals on the right hand side of equations (30
a,b) and have a reasonably accurate representation of the desired curve for $\lambda(x)$. In Arminski et al. (1979 a,b) it is
demonstrated that all three objectives can be achieved for vesicle diffusion with and without steric hindrance by the approximating function (25) which contains two adjustable parameters.
The numerical integration of equations (30 a,b) when this expression for λ is used is straight forward except for very early
times where the differential equations are singular since both
$d\delta_1/dt$ and $d\delta_2/dt$ become infinite as t^* approaches zero. This
difficulty is overcome by using a short time analytic solution
described in greater detail in Arminski et al. (1979 a) to ini-
tiate the numerical integration. One can also show analytically
that the undetermined function $A(t^*)$ in the profile (10) for the
van der Waals layer at the luminal membrane is zero for $t^* < t_1^*$
and $\alpha_1(t^*)\ell\phi$ for $t^* > t_1^*$.

Fig. 9 shows a typical solution for the evolution of the labeled free vesicle concentration profiles based on the solutions

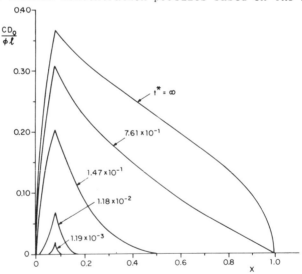

FIG. 9. Solutions to eqn. (30 a,b) for labeled free vesicles.
Loading initiated at $t^* = 0$ at luminal surface. $\lambda(x)$ based on
eqn. (25) and Ganatos et al. (7). From Arminski et al. (1).

for $\lambda(x)$ given in Ganatos et al. (7) for vesicle loading initiated at $t^* = 0$ at the luminal surface. Representative values
of the cell parameters for this figure are $\ell = 2500$ Å, $\varepsilon = 15$ Å
and a = 350 Å.

In Fig. 10 we have compared the theoretical predictions of
the theory with the time dependent labeling experiments of
Casley-Smith and Chin (3). c/c_T is the ratio of the labeled
to total free vesicle density. The solid curves are based on
the exact solutions of Ganatos et al. (7) for $\lambda(x)$ in which
the effect of the steric hindrance of attached vesicles is
neglected. These solutions provide reasonable agreement with
experiment for short time but a much poorer agreement as the
steady state is approached. (Casley-Smith and Chin state that
the 16 sec data is indicative of steady state values). The
dashed curve in the figure shows the substantial improvement in
the theoretically predicted steady state profile obtained when
$\lambda(x)$ is determined from the laboratory model experiments of
Arminski et al. (2) in which the steric hindrance of attached
vesicles is measured for several representative attached
vesicle densities. Results shown are for an hexagonal array
of attached vesicles with a mean center to center spacing of
1300 Å.

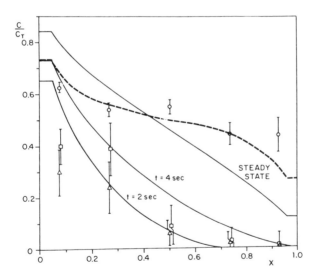

FIG. 10. Comparison of theory, Arminski et al. (2), and
experiment, Casley-Smith and Chin (3), for proportion of free
vesicles that are labeled as a function of dimensionless
distance x. Solid curves based on solution of Ganatos et al.
(7) for $\lambda(x)$. Dashed curve includes effects of steric hindrance
of attached vesicles Arminski et al. (2). Experimental data:
Δ, 2 sec; $\square$, 4 sec; o, 16 sec. Vertical bars represent ± 1
standard error.

Mechanically Enhanced Transport

The diffusional transport of plasmalemmal vesicles in the endothelial cells may be enhanced by irreversible intracellular fluid motion induced by oscillatory mechanical disturbances. In this section we outline our theoretical computation of this mechanical enhancement of vesicle transport (to be published) and correlate it with the results of experimental studies.

Since $\phi_R = P/V$, from equation (24),

$$\phi_R = \frac{Nk^d_1}{2} \left(\frac{\zeta(y)}{\zeta(1-\epsilon)}\right) \frac{1}{1 + \frac{k^d_1}{k^d_{-1}} + \frac{N_f^* \ell^2 k^d_1}{2D_o}} \tag{32}$$

It is assumed that periodic mechanical disturbances do not change N, k^d_1 or ϕ_R/ϕ, but the resulting increase in vesicle diffusion (increased D_o) causes t_D to be reduced. Since the rate of vesicle formation (k^d_{-1}) is much faster than the rate of vesicle detachment (k^d_1) and the parameter $\ell^2 k^d_1/D_o$ gives the ratio of t_D to t_a, the ratio of vesicle flux with mechanical disturbance (ϕ_R) to that in the undisturbed state (ϕ_{Ro}) can be expressed in the following equation:

$$\frac{\phi_R}{\phi_{Ro}} = \frac{1 + (N_f^* t_{Do}/2t_a)}{1 + (N_f^* t_D/2t_a)} \tag{33}$$

where t_D and t_{Do} are vesicle diffusion times in the disturbed and control states, respectively. Since N_f^* is equal to $N_{fo}t_a/N_{ao}t_{Do}$, equation (33) approaches the following limiting form, as t_D approaches 0:

$$\frac{\phi_R}{\phi_{Ro}} \rightarrow \frac{N}{N - N_{fo}} \qquad \text{as } t_D \rightarrow 0 \tag{34}$$

where N_{fo} is the free vesicle concentration in the undisturbed, control state. Our electron microscopic studies (Chien et al., unpublished observation) indicate that N_{fo} is approximately equal to 0.1 N in the endothelium of dog common carotid artery, and hence the limiting ratio ϕ_R/ϕ_{Ro} is approximately 1.1.

Experimental studies on the effect of oscillatory variations in vessel length have been carried out on isolated segments of common carotid arteries of the dog (5). The isolated segment was mounted on a rig immersed in a 0.9% NaCl bath at $37^\circ C$, and its lumen was filled with autologous serum containing ^{125}I-albumin. Experimental segments were subjected to 15 min of sinusoidal shortening in length (maximum change = 4%), and the control segments remained stationary for 15 min. After rinsing with 0.9% NaCl solution and fixation with 2% glutaraldehyde solution, the luminal diameter and ^{125}I-albumin uptake were determined in the arterial segments. The ratio of

125I-albumin uptakes per unit wall weight between the oscillated and control segments rose with increasing frequencies of oscillation to reach a plateau of 1.40 at frequencies above 5 Hz. The ratio of apparent luminal circumferences between the oscillated and control segments also increased with an increase of frequency to a plateau level of 1.30 at frequencies above 5 Hz. Therefore, at high frequencies of oscillation (above 5 Hz), there was an increase of 125I-albumin uptake of 40%, which was largely attributable to an increase in the area available for macromolecular transport as some of the endothelial cells become flattened by the oscillation. Therefore, the results are in agreement with the theoretical computation that the maximum increase in vesicle flux by periodic mechanical disturbance is only of the order of 10%.

SUMMARY

Theoretical models for the quantitative analysis of steady state and time dependent vesicle transport processes have been reviewed and correlated with experimental data. In the steady state diffusion model of Weinbaum and Caro (20), a spatially varying diffusivity is introduced to take account of the hydrodynamic and van der Waals force interactions between the vesicle and the plasmalemmal membranes. This allowed a computation of steady state concentration profile of vesicles released from each front of the endothelial cell. With the incorporation of the concept of the kinetics of vesicle attachment/detachment introduced by Rubin (14), Arminski et al. (1) have computed the steady state permeability as a function of the ratio of vesicle diffusion to attachment times. Arminski et al. (1) have also examined the time dependent behavior of labeled vesicles released from endothelial cell fronts. The computed concentration profile of the labeled free vesicles in the endothelial cell has been compared with the experimental data of Casley-Smith and Chin (3); the agreement is good if steric hindrance of vesicle attachment is included in the theoretical computation. The effect of periodic mechanical disturbance on vesicle flux has been computed and compared with the experimental results on albumin transport by arterial wall by Chien et al. (5) The results of these investigations indicate that mathematical modeling of vesicle transport in endothelial cell, in conjunction with available structural and functional data, has helped to elucidate the mechanism of transendothelial transport of macromolecules.

REFERENCES

1. Arminski, L., Weinbaum, S. and Pfeffer, R. (1979a):
    Time dependent theory for vesicular transport across
    vascular endothelium. J. Theor. Biol., in press.

2. Arminski, L., Chien, S., Pfeffer, R. and Weinbaum, S.
    (1979b): Steric hindrance effects on the time dependent
    vesicular transport of macromolecules across vascular
    endothelium. J. Theor. Biol., to be submitted.

3. Casley-Smith, J.R. and Chin, J.C. (1971): The passage
    of cytoplasmic vesicles across the endothelial and
    mesothelial cells. J. Microsc. 93:167-189, 1971.

4. Chien, S. (1978): Transport across arterial
    endothelium. In: Progress in Hemostasis and Thrombosis,
    edited by T.H. Spaet, pp. 1-36. Grune and Stratton, N.Y.

5. Chien, S., Usami, S., Fan, F.-C., Skalak, R., Weinbaum,
    S., and Caro, C.G. (1978): Effect of mechanical
    disturbances on uptake of macromolecules by the arterial
    wall. In: The Role of Fluid Mechanics in Atherogenesis,
    ed. R.M. Nerem and J.F. Cornhill, Columbus, Ohio: Ohio
    State University, pp. 16-1 to 16-4.

6. Clough, G. and Michel, C.C. (1978): Effect of albumin
    on the labeling of endothelial cell vesicles with
    ferritin. Proc. Physiol. Soc. Dec. 1978, p. 95.

7. Ganatos, P., Weinbaum, S. and Pfeffer, R. (1979): A
    strong interaction theory for the creeping motion of a
    sphere between plane parallel boundaries. Part I.
    Perdendicular motion. J. Fluid Mechanics in press.

8. Green, H.S. and Casley-Smith, J.R. (1972): Calculations
    on the passage of small vesicles across endothelial cells
    by Brownian motion. J. Theor. Biol. 35:103-111, 1972.

9. Landis, E.M. and Pappenheimer, J.R. (1963): Exchange of
    substances through the capillary walks. In: Handbook of
    Physiology; Section 2: Circulation, pp. 961-1034.
    American Physiological Society, Washington, D.C.

10. Lodish, H.F. and Rothman, J.E. (1979): The assembly of
    cell membranes. Scient. Am. 240:48-63

11. Palade GE: Fine structure of blood capillaries. J.
    Appl. Phys. 24:1424, 1953

12. Palade, G.E. and Bruns, R.R. (1968): Structural modulation of plasmalemmal vesicles. J. Cell. Biol. 37:633-649, 1968.

13. Renkin, E.M. (1978): Transport pathways through capillary endothelium. Microvasc. Res. 15:123-135.

14. Rubin, B.T. (1977): A theoretical model of the pinocytotic vesicular transport process in endothelial cells. J. Theor. Biol. 64:619-647.

15. Shea, S.M. and Bossert, W.H. (1973): Vesicular transport across endothelium: A generalized diffusion model. Microvasc. Res. 6:305-315, 1973.

16. Shea, S.M., Karnovsley, M.J. and Bossert, W.H. (1969): Vesicular transport across endothelium: Simulation of a diffusion model. J. Theor. Biol. 24:30-42, 1969.

17. Simionescu, N., Simionescu, M. and Palade, G.E. (1973): Permeability of muscle capillaries to exogenous myoglobin. J. Cell. Biol. 57:434-452.

18. Simionescu, M., Simionescu, N. and Palade, G.E. (1974): Morphometric data on the endothelium of blood capillaries. J. Cell. Biol. 60:128-152, 1974.

19. Tomlin, S.G. (1969): Vesicular transport across endothelial cells. Biochem. Biophys. Acta. 183:559-564, 1969.

20. Weinbaum, S. and Caro, C.G. (1976): A macromolecule transport model for the arterial wall and endothelium based on the ultrastructural specialization observed in electron microscopic studies. J. Fluid Mechanics 74:611-640, 1976.

This investigation was supported by Research Grants from the National Heart, Lung and Blood Institute (HL-19454) and from the National Science Foundation (ENG 78-22101).

Mathematics of Microcirculation Phenomena,
edited by J. F. Gross and A. Popel.
Raven Press, New York © 1980.

Probabalistic Solutions and Models: Oxygen Transport in the Brain Microcirculation

Duane Frederick Bruley

*Department of Chemical Engineering, Rose-Hulman Institute of Technology,
Terre Haute, Indiana 47803*

INTRODUCTION

The life scientist is primarily concerned with experimentation and the testing of hypotheses in living organisms, which represent geometrically complex heterogeneous, non-linear, interacting systems. Successes are optimized if a stable, carefully monitored and controlled model from which extraneous factors have been eliminated is available. The researcher can then vary select parameters and observe the responses, thus efficiently and quantitatively elucidating the behavior of the process. The model could be a sophisticated computerized simulation. Advances in computer technology, among these minicomputers and microprocessors, have placed greatly expanded computational power at the disposal of the biologist as well as the engineer.

The aim of the research presented here has been to develop models and solution strategies to better understand the mechanisms of neuronal survival through the simulation of the transport and reaction of oxygen in brain tissue. Specifically, the probabalistic approach has been taken to more effectively deal with the geometric complexity and the heterogeneous nature of the cerebral capillary bed.

Initial work in this field has prompted a continuing evaluation of modeling techniques. August Krogh introduced one of the earliest models in 1918--the "Krogh tissue cylinder" (FIG. 1.), and with the assistance of the Danish mathematician Erlang, obtained an analytical solution that gave quantitative values for oxygen tension in tissue (28, 29 , 30 , 31).

Through the years, improvements were made upon this original effort, the tempo of activity greatly increasing with availability of high speed electronic computers. In recent years lumped parameter models have been employed to study overall system responses such as autoregulation (4). Distributed parameter deterministic models were introduced to provide localized concentrations and to predict trends in behavior throughout the system. These were de-

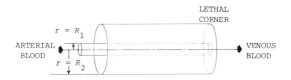

FIG. 1. Krogh tissue cylinder

rived via material balances on the Krogh tissue cylinder (5,16,36). Several other geometries have been investigated, most depending on a well ordered array of capillaries and neurons with appropriate assumptions to expedite computation (1 , 19 , 35). It has always been readily apparent that models based on such geometries and homogenous tissue were limited in the simulation of neuronal survival; yet more complex geometries presented a great obstacle to effective mathematical description, much less solution.

The necessity for simulating a realistic geometry is acutely felt, particularly by the life scientist who is intimately aware of the myriad of forms the capillary network can take. To deal with this challenge, several probabalistic simulation techniques were investigated. These include the discrete (20) and continuous (22) Monte Carlo solution of sets of deterministic, nonlinear partial differential equations describing the Krogh cylinder geometry and the stochastic physical (18) model for a single erythrocyte in a Krogh cylinder geometry. Finally an approach was developed (42) to solve the green's function in a more direct manner for each grid point throughout a three dimensional system. The model is composed of probabalistically distributed regions of convection, reaction, and oxyhemoglobin dissociation.

STOCHASTIC PROCESSES: THEORY AND APPLICATION

The theoretical development of the random walk is first presented, followed by a brief summary of the discrete and continuous process Monte Carlo methods.

Historical Development

A stochastic process is a series of random occurrences (e.g., the generation of a molecule, its motion, or its reaction) which may be a function of time. The stochastic process of chief interest here is the random motion of a particle represented as a random walk.

The concept of the random walk has long been known, but practical applications were few until the advent of high speed electronic computers.

Pearson (37) is generally credited with first formulating the problem in 1905. He formulated this concise description of the random walk:

"A man starts from a point 0 and walks 1 yard in a straight line, he then turns through any angle whatever, and walks another 1 yard in a second straight line. He repeats the process n times. I require the probability that after these n steps he is a distance r-dr from his origin 0."

Lord Rayleigh (38) demonstrated in 1889 that for a one dimensional random walk, the probability of being within a certain interval ΔR after n discrete displacements with a duration of Δt is the solution of a differential equation in the limit as Δt approaches zero.

Markov proposed in 1912 a general solution to the problem posed by Pearson (37, 23).

In 1827, the English botanist Robert Brown discovered the random motion of particles suspended in a fluid (32). However, it was not until 1905 that Albert Einstein advanced a satisfactory theoretical explanation for Brownian Motion.

Einstein (14) defined the theoretical basis for this phenomena in his monograph published in 1905. He showed that the variance of motion of a particle is

$$\bar{s}^2 = 2Dt, \tag{1}$$

where D is the diffusion coefficient; and t, time. He also showed the displacements $x(t_2) - x(t_1)$. . .$x(t_n) - x(t_n-1)$ to be mutually independent and the frequency distribution

$$p(x,t) = (\frac{1}{4\pi Dt})^{\frac{1}{2}} \exp [-(x-x_0)^2/4Dt], \tag{2}$$

(where $x-x_0$ is the displacement in time t) to be Gaussian with mean zero and to satisfy the diffusion equation

$$\frac{\partial P}{\partial t} = D \frac{\partial^2 P}{\partial x^2} \tag{3}$$

This equation is often referred to as the Fokker-Planck equation (17). From equation (1), Einstein showed that $D = 2RT/nf$ where R is the universal gas constant and n is Avagadro's Number, and f is a friction term.

In 1914 Fokker (17) related the Brownian Motion of a particle to the problem of random flight. He derived the differential equation for the transitional probability of the particle velocity and then related the differential equation to Langevin's equation of motion.

Smoluchowski (1916) (45) extended the theory of the motion of free particles to include those subject to external forces.

Langevin (1908) (32) advanced the thoery of Brownian Motion with an equation of motion for free particles (m=mass; v=velocity; F=external force):

$$m \frac{dv}{dt} = fv + F(t) \tag{4}$$

He showed that for the general case, the frequency distribution satisfied the equation

$$\frac{\partial P}{\partial t} = \frac{-1}{f} \frac{\partial (FP)}{\partial x} + \frac{\partial^2 P}{\partial x^2} \tag{5}$$

He specifically investigated the cases for which $F(x) = -a$, as for gravity; and, for $F(x) = bx$, as for elastically bound particles. The validity of the theories proposed by Einstein and Smoluchowski is limited to large values of time. Ulenbeck and Orstein (1930) (40) extended the previous work to find general frequency distributions for all time. Chandrasekhar and Doob (7 , 12) further developed this theory.

In 1931, Kolmogorov published his significant work (26) on stochastic processes. Kolmogorov derived his classic forward and backward differential equations and presented his equation which defined the Markov property. This property states that a "Markov chain" is a series of events such that each event is dependent only on the one that preceded it. Kolmogorov's work completed the theoretical foundation for the continuous parameter Markov process Monte Carlo method.

During the last years of World War II scientists and mathematicians working on the development of atomic weapons at Los Alamos needed solutions to certain very complicated integro-differential equations describing radioactive particle transport through shields (20). Unfortunately, the equations that the physicists had derived to simulate the transport process were too complicated to be solved by conventional techniques. At this time someone came up with the idea to directly simulate the transport process rather than to attempt to solve the integro-differential equations. As a charged particle approached a shieldwall, there was a probability whether it would strike a nucleus or be transmitted through the shield. If the particle struck a nucleus, there was a prabability distribution of the angle of reflection and a further probability of the particle striking another nucleus. If the probability distributions of striking a nucleus and reflection angle could be estimated, the passage of a particle through a shield could be followed until it was either reflected back, transmitted, or absorbed. The mathematicians reasoned that if the paths of a large number of particles were followed, the fraction transmitted by the shield would be an estimate of the shield's efficiency. To describe the top secret probabalistic

method for computation of shield thickness that developed from
these musings the rather transparent code name Monte Carlo was
used.   Actually the Monte Carlo method or something similar to it
was known far back in history.   An example of this is Lord Rayleigh's (38) drunkard's walk problem.   However, the method remained somewhat impractical until the development of the large
scale digital computer with its ability to make a large number of
calculations in a short period.

Because of the later arrival of the name Monte Carlo one may
find papers using this method described as employing random walks,
model sampling, drunkard's walks or the Monte Carlo method.   Perhaps the most important difference between earlier applications of
similar methods and today's work is the emphasis placed on finding
probabalistic solutions for deterministic problems.

The Monte Carlo method has been used in attacking a wide variety of problems.   Some of the problems approached by this method
are the evaluation of integrals, the passage of charged particles
through shields, the inversion of matrices, many operations research problems, and the solution of differential equations.   In
this section emphasis will be placed on the latter topic although
the others will be covered when they appear to be relevant.

Shortly after World War II as digital computers became available, papers were published that applied the Monte Carlo method to
the solution of differential equations.   A leader in the development of this method was the IBM Corporation who hosted several
computation seminars where, among other topics, the Monte Carlo
method was discussed.   Unfortunately, most of the early investigators were more concerned with programming the then new digital
computers than with explaining the problems they solved.

In 1949, the term Monte Carlo was popularized by Metropolis
and Ulam as a statistical method for the solution of complex
mathematical problems (34).   A number of papers were introduced
in 1949 (11, 41).   Perhaps the most significant was that by J. H.
Curtiss (10).   In it Curtiss gives emphasis to the use of the
Monte Carlo method in the solution of differential and difference
equations.   He derived the Monte Carlo method solution for the
following differential equation and attendant boundary conditions:

$$\beta_{11} \frac{\partial^2 U}{\partial x^2} + 2\beta_{12} \frac{\partial^2 U}{\partial x \partial y} + \beta_{22} \frac{\partial^2 U}{\partial y^2} + 2\alpha_1 \frac{\partial U}{\partial x} + 2\alpha_2 \frac{\partial U}{\partial y} = 0 \qquad (6)$$

where:

β_{11}, β_{12}, β_{22}, α_1, and α_2 are constants.

$U(x,y) = f(x,y)$, (x,y) on the boundary

The finite difference analog of Equation (6) is

$$V(x) = P_1(x,y) \ V(x+h,y) + P_2(x,y) \ V(x,y-h) + P_3(x,y)$$
$$V(x-h,y) \mp P_4(x,y) \ V(x,y+h) \mp P_5(x,y) \ V(x+h,y+h) \qquad (7)$$

where:

$$P_1(x,y) = \frac{\beta_{11} - 2\beta_{12} + 2h\alpha_1}{D}, \quad P_2(x,y) = \frac{\beta_{22} - 2\beta_{12} + 2h\alpha_2}{D},$$

$$P_3(x,y) = \frac{\beta_{11}}{D}, \quad P_4(x,y) = \frac{\beta_{22}}{D}, \quad \text{and } P_5(x,y) = \frac{2\beta_{12}}{D}$$

$$D = D(x,y) = 2\beta_{11} + 2\beta_{22} - 2\beta_{12} + 2h(\alpha_1 + \alpha_2)$$

Note that $\sum\limits_{j=1}^{5} Pj(x,y) = 1.$

He proposes the following probabalistic model for Equation (6):
A particle starts at a point (x_0,y_0) inside the region and per-
forms a random walk. The probability of a step of length h from
(x_0,y_0) to (x_0+h,y_0) is P_1; the probability of a step of length
h from (x_0,y_0) to (x_0,y_0-h) is P_2; the probability of a step of
length h from (x_0,y_0) to (x_0-h,y_0) is P_3; the probability of a
step of length h from (x_0,y_0) to (x_0,y_0+h) is P_4; and the probability of a step of length $h\sqrt{2}$ from (x_0,y_0) to (x_0+h,y_0+h) is P_5,
and the values of the dependent variable at the boundary point is
tallied. Curtiss proves that the mean value of this tally for a
large number of walks converges to the solution of Equation (6) at
the point (x_0,y_0).

A number of other works (15,22 ,24 , 27 ,33) have been achieved
since Curtiss. Further efforts have led to two separate approaches
one discrete, one continuous. The continuous Monte Carlo method
was introduced in 1960 by Chuang, Kazda, and Windeknecht (9) who
modified an analog computer for the boundary-crossing detection
of a simulated random walk.

In the hybrid solution of a continuous process Monte Carlo simulation, a noise generator supplied a series of random variables
representing the velocity of a particle's random walk. The walk
is described by a stochastic differential equation of motion such
as

$$\frac{dx}{dt} = N(t) \qquad (8)$$

where N(t) is White Gaussian noise with mean zero. In the Continuous Monte Carlo technique, these equations are generally first
order, may be nonlinear, and are related to the equation of diffusion describing the process under study. The digital portion of
the computer is employed to total results and control the logical
operations of the simulation such as selecting the response to

boundary crossings.

Development continued in this area. In 1965, Little (33) presented an extensive work describing the continuous process approach for solving linear partial differential equations, both parabolic and elliptic. Time-dependent, time-independent, homogeneous and non-homogeneous cases were also considered. Several other works have since been accomplished (6 , 21 , 24 , 25 , 27 , 33 , 44).

GREEN'S FUNCTION, THE COMMON DENOMINATOR

All of the techniques to be discussed in this work represent attempts to solve the green's function:

$$P(x,y,z,t) = \int\int\int_{a}^{b} P(x^1,y^1,z^1,t^1) \ (\tfrac{\alpha}{\pi})^{3/2} \ \exp(k\Delta t) \qquad (9)$$

$$\exp\{-\alpha(x-x^1-V_y\Delta t)^2 - \alpha(y-y^1-V_y\Delta t)^2$$

$$-\alpha(z-z^1-V_z\Delta t)^2\} \ dx^1dy^1dz^1$$

where:

$$\alpha = \frac{1}{4D\Delta t}$$

$P(x,y,z,t)$ = the solution Po_2 at (x,y,z,t)

$P(x^1,y^1,z^1,t^1)$ = the initial Po_2 throughout the region surrounding (x,y,z)

$\Delta t = t-t^1$ time increment

D = coefficient of diffusion

V = flow rate, assumed to be non-zero only in x-direction

k = first order reaction rate constant

The exponential terms represent the transition density function that the molecules at (x^1,y^1,z^1) to (x,y,z) in Δt.

Halberg, Bruley, and Knisely and Hunt and Bruley used Monte Carlo techniques whereby random walks were performed from a grid point into the surrounding tissue. For example, a one dimensional illustration of the Monte Carlo method employed by Hunt and Bruley would be as follows.

Given a one dimensional oxygen profile through a volume, a set of grid points is established. From these grid points random walks are performed. A random function generator and analog to digital converter supply the magnitude of each step. The magnitudes satisfy a Gaussian distribution determined by the coefficient of diffusivity and the size of the time step, Δt.

At the end point of each random walk, the initial condition pressure $P(x^1, t^1)$ is recorded and added to a tally. The distribution of the end points follows the exponential distribution of the equation on the preceding page.

Since the pressures obey this frequency distribution, their summation represents the integration of the product of the exponential term and the pressures throughout the surrounding region.

$$P(x_s, t_s) = \frac{\sum\limits_{i=1}^{N} P(x^1, t^1)}{N} \qquad (10)$$

where: $P(x_s, t_s)$ = the solution pressure, mm Hg

$P(s^1, t^1)$ = the initial pressure in the surrounding region at the end point of random walk i

N = total number of random walks

Chang and Bruley (8) and Groome, Bruley and Knisely (18) took the alternate approach of permitting representative oxygen molecules to diffuse through the tissue for Δt seconds.

Molecules initially within volume element i (3) are permitted to diffuse according to a Gaussian distribution for Δt. After all molecules from i have moved, the total number transferred to each of the other blocks is noted.

Here again the shift of these molecules would represent (in cumulative form) the integral of the product of the initial pressure profile and the transition density function governing the diffusion of the oxygen molecules.

This approach is distinct from those used by Halberg and Hunt in that the random walks are performed forward in time $t_{init} \rightarrow t_{final}$ versus backward from $t_{final} \rightarrow t_{init}$ as in Monte Carlo techniques.

The common denominator among the works of Halberg, Hunt, Chang, and Groome was the use of random walks to solve the green's function governing molecular motion and reaction. As well these investigators solved systems with a specific geometric configuration the Krogh Cylinder.

The primary objective of the investigation by Williford and Bruley (42) was to mathematically model the oxygen transport required for neuronal survival in a probabalistically described section of brain tissue. Specifically, the aim was to formulate and solve models incorporating distributions of capillary and neuronal activity in a more geometrically complex environment than currently employed. There are two significant advantages to this approach: first, the use of probabalistic distributions permits a more general solution than that using a specific geometric case; second, the use of a three dimensional system permits a much more sophisticated simulation than those employing the Krogh tissue cylinder.

The approach taken is to solve green's function in a more direct manner for each grid point throughout a three dimensional system. The system is composed of probabalistically distributed regions of convection, reaction and oxyhemoglobin dissociation. The solution is obtained by assuming relative homogeneity of tissue in the region of each grid point and linear oxygen profiles among all points. Each grid point is surrounded by eight octants.

Essentially the expected value of the exponential term in the green's function is used to determine the mean transition of molecules to the solution grid point from each of the eight octants (four in each hemisphere) surrounding it. This approach gives the effect of the initial pressure profile upon the new pressure at the solution point after Δt.

CASE STUDIES: THEORETICAL TECHNIQUES

Four theoretical investigations of oxygen transport in the mocrocirculation will be presented. The studies include solution by discrete Monte Carlo (Digital Computer (20)) and continuous Monte Carlo (Hybrid computer (22)) methods. Also, the stochastic physical approach (18) and the probabalistically distributed model (42) are illustrated.

The discrete and continuous Monte Carlo techniques represent probabalistic solution methods to sets of deterministic non-linear partial differential equations. The stochastic physical approach (8, 18) and probabalistically distributed model (42) do not involve deterministic equations derived from basic physical principles but do represent solutions of the green's function.

Discrete Monte Carlo

To obtain the partial differential equations describing the transport process, mass balances are made over differential volume elements in the capillary and tissue. At the interface between them it is assumed that there is no resistance to mass transfer and that Fick's first law is applicable in both the capillary and tissue. Some of the more important assumptions made in the derivation follow:

1. The Krogh tissue cylinder geometry is applicable.
2. The reaction between chemically bound oxygen in the erythrocytes and dissolved oxygen in the plasma is so rapid that the two are at equilibrium, and the relationship between them may be expressed by ψ, the oxygen dissociation curve. Furthermore, ψ is assumed to be a function of the oxygen partial pressure only.
3. The supply of chemically bound oxygen is distributed homogeneously throughout the capillary.
4. The blood velocity profile is flat.
5. At the blood-tissue interface there is no resistance to mass transfer, and transport is by diffusion only.

6. Oxygen consumption in the tissue cylinder is a con-
    stant-consumption zero-order reaction.

The equation describing oxygen transport in the capillary is:

$$\frac{\partial P}{\partial t} = \frac{D_1}{[1 + \frac{N}{C_1} \frac{d\psi}{dP}]} [\frac{\partial^2 P}{\partial r^2} + \frac{1}{r} \frac{\partial P}{\partial r} + \frac{\partial^2 P}{\partial z^2}] - v \frac{\partial P}{\partial z} \tag{11}$$

At the interface the following two equations apply:

$$P_i \bigg| \text{ capillary } = P_i \bigg| \text{ tissue} \tag{12}$$

$$D_1 c_1 \frac{\partial P}{\partial r} \bigg| \text{ capillary } = D_2 c_2 \frac{\partial P}{\partial r} \bigg| \text{ tissue} \tag{13}$$

The following equation is derived for oxygen transport and consumption in the tissue cylinder:

$$\frac{\partial P}{\partial r} = D_2 [\frac{\partial^2 P}{\partial r^2} + \frac{1}{r} \frac{\partial P}{\partial r} + \frac{\partial^2 P}{\partial z^2}] - \frac{A}{c_2} \tag{14}$$

These equations are solved simultaneously with the following
boundary conditions:

$$\frac{\partial P}{\partial r} = 0, \; r = 0, \; 0 < z < L, t \geq 0$$

$$\frac{\partial P}{\partial r} = 0, \; r = R_2, \; 0 \leq z < 1, \; t \geq 0$$

$$\frac{\partial P}{\partial z} = 0, \; z = L, \; 0 \leq r < R_2, \; t \geq 0$$

$$\frac{\partial P}{\partial z} = 0, \; z = 0, \; R_1 < r < R_2, \; t \geq 0$$

$$P = P(r), \; z = 0, \; 0 < r < R_1, \; t \geq 0$$
$$P = P(r,z), \; 0 \leq z \leq L, \; 0 \leq r \leq R_2, \; t = 0$$

To obtain unsteady-state solutions, it was decided to use the
Monte Carlo method to solve the above system of equations. The
Monte Carlo method has the advantage that it is possible to obtain the solution to a set of partial differential equations at
one point in space only. Conventional techniques obtain the solution for all points in space at once. Therefore, it was proposed
to solve for oxygen partial pressure at the lethal corner only,
for upsets in arterial oxygen partial pressure, and for flow rate.
    To proceed with the solution, the partial derivatives are re-
placed by their finite difference approximations. For reasons

that will be explained later it will be generally possible to use only first-order approximations for the Monte Carlo method. When these substitutions have been made and the results solved for $P(r,z,t+1)$, Equations 11, 12, 13, and 14 become

$$P(r,z,t+1) = P(r+h_1,z,t) \ [\frac{K\ell}{h_1^2} + \frac{K\ell}{2rh_1}]$$

$$+ \ P(r-h_1,z,t) \ [\frac{K\ell}{h_1^2} - \frac{K\ell}{2rh_1}] \ + \ P(r,z+k,t) \ [\frac{K\ell}{K^2}]$$

$$+ \ P(r,z-k,t) \ [\frac{K\ell}{K^2} + \frac{\nu\ell}{K}] \qquad (15)$$

$$+ \ P(r,z,t) \ [1 - \frac{2K\ell}{h_1^2} - \frac{2K\ell}{K^2} - \frac{\nu\ell}{K}]$$

where

$$K = [\frac{D_1}{1+N \ \frac{d\Psi}{C_1 \ dP}}]$$

$$P(r,z,t) = P(r+h_2,z,t) \ [\frac{\frac{D_2 C_2}{h_2}}{\frac{D_1 C_1}{h_1} + \frac{D_2 C_2}{h_2}}]$$

$$+ \ P(r-h_1,z,t) \ [\frac{\frac{D_1 C_1}{h_1}}{\frac{D_1 C_1}{h_1} + \frac{D_2 C_2}{h_2}}] \qquad (16)$$

$$P(r,z,t+1) = P(r+h_2,z,t) \ [\frac{D_2\ell + D_2\ell}{h_2^2} \quad \frac{}{2rh_2}]$$

$$+ P(r+h_1 z,t) \left[\frac{\frac{D_2 \ell}{2}}{h_2^2} - \frac{\frac{D_2 \ell}{2}}{2rh_2} \right] + P(r,z+K,t) \left[\frac{\frac{D_2 \ell}{2}}{K^2} \right]$$

$$+ P(r,z-k,t) \left[\frac{\frac{D_2 \ell}{2}}{K^2} \right] \qquad (17)$$

$$+ P(r,z,t) \left[1 - \frac{\frac{2D_2 \ell}{2}}{h_2^2} - \frac{\frac{2D_2 \ell}{2}}{K^2} \right] - \frac{A\ell}{C_2}$$

These equations may be written in the general form

$$P_o = \sum_{i=1}^{5} Pr_i P_i - C$$

where C is a constant either equal to zero or $(A \cdot \ell/C_2)$ for this case.

For the Monte Carlo method Equations 15, 16, and 17 must be interpreted as probabilistic difference equations in which the coefficients of the various P_i's are one-step transition probabilities from point P_o to P_i. Note that, reassuringly, the sum of the probabilities is equal to one for each equation. Since probabilities are defined only for the interval between zero and one, h_1, h_2, k, and ℓ must be chosen such that no probability falls outside this range. It is this limitation also which prohibits the use of higher-ordered finite difference approximations.

To obtain a solution to this system of partial differential equations at a point r_0, Z_0 and time, $T = N\ell$, a particle is allowed to begin a walk at this point stepping from mesh point to mesh point. At each step in the walk the particle must satisfy the appropriate difference equation. At r_0, Z_0 a random number Q is obtained which is uniformly distributed between zero and one. If $0 \leq Q \leq Pr_1$, the particle takes a step from point 0 to point 1. If $Pr_1 \leq Q \leq Pr_1 + Pr_2$, the particle steps from point 0 to point 2, and similar expressions hold for the rest of the probability intervals. Note that each step in space is also a step backwards in time from t + 1 to t.

For the walk a tally is started at zero, and at each step in the walk a quantity C is subtracted from the tally. The walk is allowed to continue for N steps if no boundary is reached, after which it will be at some position in the region and time will be zero. Since there is an initial-condition pressure mesh available, the appropriate differential equation is identically satisfied, and the walk is terminated. The value of the initial pressure at the final point reached is added to the tally which is an estimate

for the value of the pressure at the starting point of the walk
and time $N\ell$. However, the accuracy of this estimate will be quite
poor, but to make an improvement it is only necessary to make
additional walks from the same starting point and use the mean
value of the tallies as an estimate for the solution. The proba-
ble difference between this estimate and the true solution will
decrease as the reciprocal of the square root of the number of
walks completed.

If a boundary point is reached at some point during a walk, a
different procedure will have to be followed depending on the type
of boundary condition. At a boundary point where the value of the
dependent variable-oxygen pressure in this case-is given, the
partial differential equation is identically satisfied for all
values of time. Therefore, when such a boundary is reached, the
walk is terminated, and the value of the dependent variable is
added to the tally. For a boundary where the derivative vanishes
(i.e., $\partial P/\partial x = 0$) the particle is reflected back into the interior
with probability one. Furthermore, it has been stated that for
the more general boundary condition

$$Pr_1 f(B) + Pr_2 (\partial f/\partial x) = 0$$

where $f(B)$ is the value of the dependent variable at the boundary
and

$$Pr_1 + Pr_2 = 1$$

Pr_1 is the probability of being reflected and Pr_2 is the probability of being absorbed.

An efficient method for obtaining a transient solution at one
point in space utilizes the fact that the Monte Carlo analog of a
partial differential equation with time invarient coefficients is
a stationary random process. Suppose a solution is desired for
time from 0 to $T = N\ell$. An interval n is chosen for which individual values will be calculated. A walk is begun at the point
where a solution is desired and allowed to continue for n steps
keeping the tally as before. The initial condition value of the
dependent variable at the last point reached is added to the tally
to obtain an estimate of the dependent variable at time n. However, since the process is stationary, the n steps completed can
also serve for the time interval 2n to n. In this manner an
estimate for the dependent variable at time 2n can be made by continuing the walk for only n more steps. But, the tally must be
continued from the value reached before the dependent variable is
added. This process may be repeated over and over until in $\geq$ N,
where i is the number of points for which a solution is obtained.
By using this technique a large saving of computational time can
be achieved.

The Monte Carlo method is directly applicable to linear partial

differential equations only. For nonlinear partial differential
equations the one-step transition probabilities will be a function
of the dependent variable. Since values for the dependent variable are what one is trying to determine, they will not be available. However, a method has been developed which will enable one
to approximate the solution of nonlinear partial differential
equations to any degree of accuracy which is desirable. The
differential analog of a nonlinear partial differential equation
may be written:

$$P_o = \sum_{i=1}^{5} Pr_i(P_o)P_i + C \qquad (18)$$

   For a small time increment the pressure mesh will not change
greatly from the initial-condition pressure values. Therefore, if
the initial values are used in calculating the one-step transition
probabilities, there will be little error. Using this technique
a whole new pressure mesh may be calculated for the small time
increment. Then, the new mesh may be used to calculate a mesh
for another small increment. In this manner a complete time
history for the whole space may be calculated with little error.
Unfortunately, if this technique is used, it will be necessary to
obtain a transient solution for the whole mesh, and one of the
advantages of the Monte Carlo method will be lost. However, this
technique will be invaluable for otherwise insoluble partial
differential equations.
   To obtain transient solutions for the lethal corner two
methods were used. The first technique involved a linearization
of Ψ.

$$\Psi = K_1 + K_2 P$$
$$d\Psi/dP = K_2 \qquad (19)$$

Equation 19 was substituted into Equation 15 and solutions were
obtained for step changes in arterial oxygen partial pressure and
capillary blood flow rate. A disadvantage of this linearization
is that it is necessary to make an a priori estimate of K_2, and
no precise method is available for this purpose. To overcome this
limitation a second method was developed which is an extension of
the technique proposed for nonlinear partial differential
equations. In this method the initial-condition pressure mesh
was used to calculate one-step transition probabilities for all
values of time, even for long time periods and large changes in
oxygen partial pressure. This technique will necessarily introduce some error; it amounts to a stepwise linearization of the
capillary equation, but no a priori estimates need be made, and a
solution can be obtained for the lethal corner only.

With Ψ represented by,

$$\Psi = \frac{KP^m}{1 + KP^m}$$

thus

$$\frac{d\Psi}{dP} = \frac{KmP^{m-1}}{(1 + KP^m)^2} \qquad (20)$$

This expression was substituted into Equation 15, and solutions were obtained for upsets in arterial oxygen partial pressure and capillary blood flow rate.

A serious disadvantage of the Monte Carlo method is the large number of walks required to obtain a sufficiently accurate solution. The following formula has been suggested for the number of walks required for n decimal places of accuracy with 0.95 probability:

$$N = 4 \times 10^{2n}(B-A)^2 \qquad (21)$$

where N is the number of walks and B and A are the maximum and minimum values of the dependent variable. As one can readily see a very large number of walks will be required for an accurate solution. For all simulations in this work 500 walks were made. To reduce the number of walks necessary for a given accuracy, many variance reduction methods have been developed. Although none of these methods has been used in this study, it is felt that successful application of variance reduction techniques is the key to reducing Monte Carlo computation time. For this problem importance sampling appears very promising.

Nomenclature

A = maximum value of dependent variable

B = minimum value of dependent variable

C = constant

c_1 = oxygen solubility coefficient for blood, cc_{O_2}/cc blood-mm Hg

c_2 = oxygen solubility coefficient for tissue, cc_{O_2}/cc blood-mm Hg

D_1 = oxygen diffusivity in blood, cm^2/sec

D_2 = oxygen diffusivity in tissue, cm^2/sec

h_1,h_2 = finite difference in r-direction, cm

k = finite difference in z-direction, cm

t = time finite difference, sec

L = length of Krogh tissue cylinder, cm

N = combined oxygen capacity of blood, cc O_2/cc blood

P = oxygen partial pressure, mm Hg

P_1 = oxygen partial pressure at interface, mm Hg

P_r = one-step transition probability

r = radial direction, cm

R_1= radius of capillary, cm
R_2= radius of tissue cylinder, cm
t = time, sec
v = velocity, cm/sec
x = distance, cm
z = axial distance, cm
  = fractional saturation of hemoglobin with combined oxygen-oxygen dissociation curve
P_0= point 0
P_1= point 1

Continuous Monte Carlo

Since the name Monte Carlo was first popularized as a statistical method for solving mathematical problems, both discrete and continuous variations of the method have been developed. The first application of the continuous Monte Carlo method involved the improvement of an analog computer for detecting the boundary-crossings of a simulated random walk. Little (33) presented a full description of the continuous approach to the solution of linear partial differential equations including parabolic and elliptic equaitons, time-dependent and time-independent equations, and homogeneous and nonhomogeneous equations. Until now, no one has attempted to use the Monte Carlo method to account for non-linearities in differential equations; however, this work presents a modification which can handle the nonlinear case.

The nonlinear Monte Carlo technique is applied to differential equations defined on an open bounded region with a closed boundary. (The same set of equations as presented for the discrete case is used.) An open bounded region is a region not extending to infinity and is a separate entity from the boundary. The open bounded region is divided into a discrete mesh; a solution can be found at any mesh point by the Monte Carlo method. In the solution of nonlinear time-dependent equations, the initial condition of time zero is satisfied by the steady-state solution of the mesh points at time zero. Furthermore, any nonlinear coefficient is approximated at time zero by substituting the steady-state solution values into its nonlinear function.

The continuous Monte Carlo method can provide a solution for each desired mesh point at a time which is a small time increment Δt from the time of the previous solution mesh. Essentially, the technique involves random walking backward for a Δt period (t_s to $t_s-\Delta t$, in the first step) for each mesh point to be solved for at t_s. After the entire mesh is computed at t_s, the nonlinear coefficient is updated by substituting values just calculated at t_s, and, if iteration is unnecessary, the solution can now be advanced to time t_s+ t by random walking backward to time t_s. Thus, an entire mesh may be updated in time using only the previous solution mesh. The solution may be stopped at any moment in time but is truly complete only when the next steady state is reached.

As described, the nonlinear coefficient is continually updated

by approximation from the mesh values of the previous solution.
The correctness of the assumption that the nonlinear coefficient
is time-independent during Δt may be checked by using a different
Δt and/or iterating using an average value of the mesh-point solutions obtained before and at the end of Δt. The nonlinear coefficient, though assumed time-independent during Δt, is dependent
upon position in the bounded region.

The uniqueness of the Monte Carlo method of calculating single-
point solutions allows freedom in choosing locations of the mesh
points. In addition, instead of producing Monte Carlo solutions
at every mesh point, mesh points may be selected and the remaining
mesh points can be approximated from the Monte Carlo solutions of
the surrounding mesh points. Judicious selection of the mesh
points reduces the computation time.

Stable random noise signals are required for accurate Monte
Carlo solutions. A random-noise generating technique was used to
transform a low-quality noise source from a thyratron tube into
two stable random-noise signals. The noise signals were observed
to be uncorrelated at time lags greater than 0.02 milliseconds,
and accordingly Δt, the time period of the random walk, exceeded
the noise signal's uncorrelation time lag by at least a factor of
one hundred.

As with any new application or modification of an established
technique, the merits of the newly developed method should be explained. The following discussion attempts to do so. As the
method-of-lines solution of the oxygen transport model is considered the best available at the present time, a favorable com-
parision with the Monte Carlo results would lend credence to the
nonlinear technique.

The solution to the nonlinear time-dependent equations confirms
the merits of the nonlinear Monte Carlo method. For step change
in arterial oxygen partial pressure, both methods indicate a new
lethal corner oxygen partial pressure near 12 mm Hg. This is important, since the nonlinearity severely affects the value at
which the transient response levels out. On the other hand, the
reason for discrepancy during the transient period is unknown and
cannot be attributed to the size of the time increment since two
different time increments produced the same end result. The close-
ness of the solutions for two time increments using 1000 random
walks shows that iterative correction is unnecessary.

A major consideration is the reduction of computation time;
hence, the number of random walks was lowered from 1000 to 400
with no apparent change of accuracy. Unfortunately, even with
this economization, the computation time was 56 minutes on a PDP
15/EAI 680 hybrid computing system.

On the positive side, with the establishment of the nonlinear
Monte Carlo method, improvements in the hardware, in the frequency
response of the noise generator and the analog computer, and in
the software (e.g., coding in machine language instead of
FORTRAN IV) should reduce the computation time considerably. Thus
the nonlinear Monte Carlo method is a powerful technique for the
solution of sophisticated mathematical models and can reduce sol-

ution times for nonlinear time-dependent partial differential e-
quations.

Stochastic Physical Method

Based on the "Krogh tissue cylinder" a coupled set of nonlinear partial differential equations describing the transport of
oxygen in the brain microcirculation have been presented. In de-
riving the equations it was assumed that (1) equilibrium exists
between the dissolved oxygen and hemoglobin; i.e., the oxygen dissociation curve serves as a reaction curve, (2) resistance at the
capillary-tissue interface is negligible, and (3) blood and tissue
are homogeneous phases.

As is evident from the set of coupled equations, predicting
oxygen levels is a formidible task, even under steady-state conditions. To simplify this, while at the same time affording a
more basic model, the following stochastic model has been developed. This model does not involve solving the deterministic model,
but instead is based on the assumption that oxygenation of the
brain can be described by simulating the activity of only one e-
rythrocyte and the oxygen molecules which surround it.

Oxygen is transferred in the capillary by bulk flow and molecular diffusion, with gradients in both the axial and radial directions. The simulation procedure consists of displacing each oxygen molecule a distance $v_x \Delta t$ and then using three Gaussianly distributed random numbers to determine the final position. In the
three-dimensional case the net displacements during the time interval Δt are:

$$x = x' + \int_x^b (R_n) + v_x \Delta t, \qquad (22)$$

$$y = y' + \int_y^b (R_n) \qquad , \qquad (23)$$

$$z = z' + \int_z^b (R_n) \qquad , \qquad (24)$$

and, for the erythrocyte,

$$x_e = x'_e + v_x \Delta t \qquad , \qquad (25)$$

where it has been assumed that bulk flow is in the x-direction
only. In the case of three-dimensional flow, i.e., the bolus
flow, the velocity field required as an input to the convective
step can be determined by a numerical solution of the Navier
Stokes equations.

At the capillary entrance the number of oxygen molecules n_0,
surrounding the erythrocyte is determined and is chosen as the
basis: n_0 molecule exert a partial pressure P_B within a volume V_B.
Erythrocytes are biconcave discs approximately 8 microns in diameter, with the rim of the disc being thicker (2 microns) than the
center (1 micron). The effective volume V_B was chosen based on a
cylindrical radius of 2.5 microns, i.e., capillary radius, and a
cylindrical length of 1 micron, the thickness of an erythrocyte at
its center. The effect of the erythrocyte volume on the movement

of oxygen was assumed negligible, Since the solubility is defined
as

$$S_o{}^b = \frac{C_o{}^b}{P_o{}^b} \tag{26}$$

where $C_o{}^b$ and $P_o{}^b$ are the concentration of oxygen in the blood and
the partial pressure of dissolved oxygen in the blood, respectively
a pseudo-solubility is calculated as

$$S_o{}^b = \frac{\eta_o/V_B}{P_B} \tag{27}$$

Under normal conditions P_B is 95 mm Hg.

Once the convective step is completed, the number of oxygen
molecules η_o within the volume V_B surrounding the erythrocyte is
determined. Since the oxygen carried on an erythrocyte is chemically bound to the hemoglobin, the fractional saturation ψ can be
thought of as the ratio of the number of hemoglobin sites filled
(N_f) to the total number of hemoglobin sites available at saturation (N_s). Thus,

$$\psi = \frac{N_f}{N_s} \tag{28}$$

and the change in ψ is a direct measure of the number of oxygen
molecules bound to the erythrocyte for some change $\Delta\psi$ in the
fractional saturation of the erythrocyte.

Assuming equilibrium to exist between the oxygen dissolved in
the plasma and the oxygen bound to the erythrocyte, the following
relations must be observed:

$$P_o = \frac{(\eta + N_r)/V_B}{S_o{}^b} \tag{30}$$

$$\psi = \frac{\theta^3 + b - 1}{\theta^4 + b - 1} \tag{31}$$

where θ is given by equation (6), and

$$N_r = -N_s(\psi - \psi_i), \tag{32}$$

where η is the number of oxygen molecules surrounding the erythrocyte before any oxygen is released by or absorbed onto the erythrocyte, and ψ_i is the previous erythrocyte saturation value. From

the above set of equations (equations 30, 31 and 32) the numbers of oxygen molecules released from the red blood cell can be determined. Since η, S_o^b, V_B, N_s, and ψ_i are known, there are three equations and three unknowns (P, ψ, and N_r). A modified Fibonacci search routine is used to converge on the partial pressure P. Once the oxygen tension is known, the fractional saturation can be found (equation 31) and the number of oxygen molecules released determined using equation 32. The positions of the released molecules are uniformly distributed within the volume V_B around the erythrocyte center.

The deterministic models were developed with the assumption that oxygen diffused freely across the capillary wall. Since the capillary wall is approximately 0.5 microns thick, as compared with a capillary radius of 2.5 microns, membrane resistance may be significant. Permeability effects can be readily incorporated into the stochastic model in the following manner. Let P_m denote the capillary wall permeability such that

$$0 \leq P_m \leq 1 \tag{33}$$

where the lower limit ($P_m=0$) represents a capillary wall of infinite permeability and the upper ($P_m=1$) is a completely impermeable membrane. A uniformly distributed random number R_n between zero and one is generated and compared to P_m. If $R_n > P_m$, the particle is allowed to pass across the capillary wall into the tissue; otherwise, it is reflected back into the capillary. To account for the finite thickness of the capillary wall, an inert region of approximately 0.5μ should be included. The treatment of this third phase offers some problems for the deterministic model, but can readily be handled with the proposed stochastic model.

Oxygen travels in the tissue by molecular diffusion only, with gradients existing in both the radial and axial directions. As in the capillary, the diffusion process is governed by the Gaussian distribution function. For three-dimensions, the net displacements during the time interval Δt are

$$x = x' + \int_x^t (R_n), \tag{34}$$

$$y = y' + \int_y^t (R_n), \tag{35}$$

and

$$z = a' + \int_z^t (R_n) \tag{36}$$

Following movement by diffusion, the next step in the simulation is to determine if the molecule has been consumed by chemical reaction in the time interval Δt. Since previous investigators have assumed a constant oxygen consumption rate to be valid under normal conditions, several techniques were tried in simulating the zero-order reaction.

For a zero-order reaction the probability density was found to be

$$P_x(t) = \frac{(kt)^{x_o-x}}{(x_o-x)!} e^{-kt} \tag{37}$$

and the expected number of molecules reacting in the time interval Δt is

$$E[N(\Delta t)] = k\Delta t, \tag{38}$$

where k is the zero-order rate constant. A tubular plug flow reactor was simulated by removing $k\Delta t$ molecules from the system for each stochastic step, and these results were then extended to the capillary-tissue system.

It is known that, for a Markov pure-jump process, the waiting time τ until a particle reacts is exponentially distributed:

$$P(\tau \leq t) = 1-e^{-\mu t}, \tag{39}$$

where $P(\tau \leq t)$ is the distribution function for τ. Using a set of exponentially distributed random numbers, τ was generated, and the particle was allowed to move until $t \geq \tau$, at which time it was deleted from the system.

Since the reaction mechanism within the tissue has not been positively established, it was decided to attempt the simulation assuming a first-order reaction. For a single particle, the probability of reaction is given by Wyman and Kosten (43) as

$$P_r = e^{-k\Delta t}. \tag{40}$$

In carrying out the simulation a uniformly distributed random number R_n is generated and compared to P_r. If $R_n > P_r$, the molecule is said to have reacted and is deleted from the system; otherwise the molecule continues its random walk.

This work was intended to develop an initial stochastic model which is simple and versatile, affording a more fundamental description of the oxygenation of the brain microcirculation while simultaneously avoiding the mathematical complexities inherent in the numerical solution of the deterministic model. The stochastic model as presented has one basic assumption: oxygen partial pressure can be obtained through the simulation of only one erythrocyte and the oxygen molecules surrounding it. This is an initial assumption with plans to examine multierythrocyte systems. The model does agree well with existing deterministic results and available experimental data for capillary space-average oxygen tensions. Although more work is still required before adequate tissue results are available, the proposed stochastic model does have considerable potential in its extension to complex anatomical patterns and multicomponent systems.

Probabalistically Distributed Model

This approach utilizes the fact that for the localized regions of relatively constant diffusivity, convection and reaction rate about each grid point, the mean transition can be calculated from these parameters and the time step. Consider the Green's function defining a one dimensional case.

The exponential terms represent a density function (continuous probability curve). Now consider the normal probability frequency function $f(x)$ in one variable with mean μ and variance σ^2, or the univariate normal:

$$f(x) = \frac{1}{\sigma(2\pi)^{1/2}} \exp\ [\frac{-(x-\mu)^2}{2\sigma^2}] \text{ is analogous to } \sqrt{2D\Delta t}$$

and μ to $-V_x\Delta t$, where $x = 0.0$.   (41)

The Monte Carlo techniques discussed previously use a series of random walks to create a sample of endpoints in the region about each grid point. These endpoints are distributed normally with respect to the point of initiation. Initial values at these points were then tallied to solve for the solution grid point value. Since the endpoints are distributed normally, the summation of pressures is implicitly the integral of the product of pressure and transition probability.

Thus

$$P_n(F_s t_s) = \frac{1}{n}\ \sum_{i=1}^{n}\ P_i(F_o,t_o) + kT_{F_s,t_s}$$ (42)

where:

P_n = the solution, dependent variable (Po_2) at the solution point F_s and time t_s

n = number of random walks

P_i = initial condition at initial point F_o and time t

k = zero order reaction rate constant

T_{F_s,t_s} = the expected (average) time for the random walks

The method presented here calculates the mean these random walks would have as a result of the tally under the old method. Consider a one dimensional case with diffusion and zero order reaction. The oxygen tension profile would be a single line passing through the solution point, X_s. The solution Green's function will be:

$$P(x_s,t_s) = \int_a^b P(x^1,t^1)\ (\tfrac{\alpha}{\pi})^{1/2}$$

$$\exp\ [-\alpha\{x-(x^1+v_x\Delta t)\}^2]\ dx + k\Delta t$$ (43)

Here, again, the second exponential function represents the

transition probability or the conditional density function:

$$f(x_s, t_s \mid x^1, t^1) \tag{44}$$

In words: given that a molecule(s) is at x^1 at time t^1, the probability that this molecule(s) will move to x_s at t_s is equal to the term $f(x_s, t_s \mid x_s^1, t^1)$.

Now consider the region between the solution grid point and the first grid point to its right. If a large set of random walks are initiated from the solution grid point, the endpoints will yield a smooth normal density function. At the end point of the ith random walk, P_i, the oxygen tension (mm Hg) is:

$$P_i = P_a + [\frac{P_b - P_a}{b-a}] * [x_i - x_a] \tag{45}$$

$$= k_1 + k_2 x_i$$

$$k_1 = P_a - x_a [\frac{P_b - P_a}{b-a}]; \quad k_2 = [\frac{P_b - P_a}{b-a}]$$

It has been shown that the solution may be formulated either from the results of a series of random walks or analytically. The latter is the approach adopted here. As previously mentioned the essential validity of this method was substantiated by a one dimensional simulation, even though it proved too susceptible to error to use as a solution technique.

The approach employed here is to use the method outlined in three dimensions and solve the following brain tissue model.

The tissue model consists of a three dimensional region 77 x 77 microns square and 140 microns in length. Within the system is a set of grid points, 11 x 11 x 20, laid out in cartesian coordinates. Each point (i,j,k) is surrounded by eight octants and at the corners of these a total of twenty-five other grid points.

As for the one dimensional case one wishes to determine the pressure at the mean vector. In the case of the three dimensional system the spherical distribution is divided among eight octants. The object is to determine the pressure at the endpoint vector. This vector represents the summation of all the individual random walk endpoint vectors which exist in the octant. Since the profile among grid points has been assumed linear, one can determine the pressure at any point within each octant by a triple linear interpolation. The solution at each grid point then becomes the average of P_7's for the eight octants which surround the grid point. Subtracting a reaction term yields the most general form of the solution equation for points in the tissue interior.

The solution at each grid point becomes an algebraic equation of the initial grid point pressures surrounding the solution grid point.

The computer executes a series of Do loops for each type of

point (face, corner, edge, etc.). Δt is on the order of 0.001 seconds thus requiring several thousand time steps. However, the calculation is very simple, consisting of sets of summations within algebraic equations, and involve minimal approximation due to the linearized oxygen tension profile between adjacent points. The consideration of heterogeneously distributed parameters with nonsymmetric boundaries thus provides a more realistic simulation of the microcirculation.

References

1. Akmal, K., Bruley, D. F., Banchero, N., Artigue, R. and Moloney, W. (1978): Multi-Capillary Model for Oxygen Transport to Skeletal Muscle. In: Oxygen Transport to Tissue-III, edited by I. A. Silver, M. Erecinska, and H. I. Bicher, pp. 139-147. Plenum Publishing Corporation.
2. Artigue, R. S., Bruley, D. F. (To Be Published). Oxygen and Carbon Dioxide Transport in Human Brain: Effect of the Mass Transfer Coefficient of the Red Blood Cell. Rose-Hulman Institute of Technology, Terre Haute, Indiana.
3. Bruley, D. F., Groome, L., Hunt, D. H., Bicher, H. I., and Knisely, M. (1975): Predicting Oxygen Supply to Brain Tissue Using a Pseudo Dynamic Model Simulation Technique. Bibl. Anat. 13:139-140.
4. Bruley, D. F., Bicher, H. I., Reneau, D. D., and Knisely, M.H. (1971): Autoregulatory Phenomena Related to Cerebral Tissue Oxygenation. Advances in Bioengineering, CEP Symposium Series 114. 67:195-201.
5. Bruley, D. F. (1972): New Results on Oxygen Transport in Capillary Tissues. AIChE Journal. 18:669.
6. Bugliarello, G., Hsiao, G. C. (1970): A Mathematical Model of the Flow in the Axial Plasmatic Gaps of the Smaller Vessels. Biorhealogy. 7:5-36.
7. Chandrasekar, S. (1943): Stochastic Problems in Physics and Astronomy. Reviews of Modern Physics. 15:1.
8. Chang, C. L. and Bruley, D. F. (1975): Quantitative Studies of Brain Microcirculation. First World Congress on Microcirculation, Toronto, Canada.
9. Chuang, K., Kazda, L. F., and Windeknecht, T. (1960): Stochastic Method of Solving Partial Differential Equations Using an Electronic Analog Computer. Project Michigan Report 2900-91-T. Willow Run Laboratories, University of Michigan.
10. Curtiss, J. H. (1949): Sampling Methods Applied to Differential and Difference Equations. Proceedings of a Seminar on Scientific Computation: IBM Corporation, New York.
11. Donsker, M. D. and Kac, M. (1950): A Sampling Method for Determining the Lowert Eigenvalue and the Principal Eigenfunction of Schrodinger's Equation. J. of Research, National Bureau of Standards. 44:551-557.
12. Doob, J. L. (1942): American Math. Monthly. 59:648.

13. Edwards, K. H. and Khana, R. R. (1970). Feasibility Study of Monte Carlo Modelling Techniques for Distributed-Parameter Systems, Parts 1 and 2. Proc. IEEE. 117:2227.

14. Einstein, A. (1956): Investigations on the Theory of the Brownian Movement. Dover Publications, New York.

15. Ehrlich, L. W. (1959): Monte Carlo Solutions of Boundary Value Problems Involving the Difference Analogue of $\partial^2 u/\partial x^2 + \partial^2 u/\partial y^2 + K/y \; \partial u/\partial y = 0$. J. Assoc. for Computing Machinery 6:204.

16. Fletcher, J. E. (1973): A Mathematical Model of the Unsteady Transport of Oxygen to Tissues in the Microcirculation. Advances in Experimental Medicine and Biology. 37B:819-825.

17. Fokker, A. D. (1914): Ann. d. Physik. 43:812.

18. Groome, L. J., Bruley, D. F., and Knisely, M. H. (1976): A Stochastic Model for the Transport of Oxygen to the Brain. Advances in Experimental Medicine and Biology. 75:267-277

19. Grunewald, W. (1973): Method of Comparison of Calculated and Measured Oxygen Distruibution. Oxygen Supply, edited by M. Kessler, D. Bruley, L. Clark, Jr., D. Lubbers, I. Silver, and J. Strauss, pp. 5-17. Strauss, Urban & Schwarzenberg, Munchen.

20. Halberg, M., Bruley, D. F., and Knisely, M. H. (1970): Simulating Oxygen Transport in the Microcirculation by Monte Carlo Methods. Simulation. 15(5):206-212.

21. Handler, H. (1967): Monte Carlo Solution of Partial Differential Equations Using a Hybrid Computer. IEEE Transactions on Electronic Computers. ED-16:603.

22. Hunt, D. H. and Bruley, D. F. (1978): A Nonlinear Monte Carlo Simulation: Oxygen Transport in the Brain. Simulation Jan.:17-27.

23. Hoel, P. G., Port, S. C., and Stone, C. J. (1972): Introduction to Stochastic Processes. Houghton Mifflin Company, Boston.

24. Johnson, E. L. (1969): A Variance Reduction Technique for the Continuous Random Walk Solution of LaPlace's Equation. Unpublished Ph.D. Siddertation, University of Kansas, Lawrence.

25. Johnson, E. L. (1970): A Variance Reduction Technique for Hybrid Computer Generated Random Walk Solutions of Partial Differential Equations. Proceedings-Spring Joint Computer Conference, p. 19

26. Kolmogorov, A. (1931): Uber die Analytischen Methoden in der Wahrscheinlichkeitsrechnung. Mathematische Annalen. 104:415.

27. Korn, G. A. (1965): Hybrid Computer Monte Carlo Techniques. Simulation. 5:234.

28. Krogh, A. (1919): The Rate of Diffusion of Gases Through Animal Tissues with Some Remarks on the Coefficient of Invasion J. Physiol. 52:391-408.

29. Krogh, A. (1919): The Number and Distribution of Capillaries in Muscles with Calculations of the Oxygen Pressure Head Necessary for Supplying the Tissue. J. Physiol. 52:409-415.

30. Krogh, A. (1918-1919): The Supply of Oxygen to the Tissues and the Regulations of the Capillary Circulation. J. Physiol 52:457-474.
31. Krogh, A. (1922): The Anatomy and Physiology of Capillaries Yale University Press, New Haven, Conn.
32. Langevin, P. (1908): On the Theory of Brownian Movement. Compte Rendus. 147:530.
33. Little, W. D. (1966): Hybrid Computer Solutions of Partial Differential Equations by Monte Carlo Methods. Proceedings Fall Joint Computer Conference, p. 181
34. Metropolis, N. and Ulam, S. (1949): The Monte Carlo Method. J. Amer. Stat. Assoc. 44:335.
35. Metzger, H. (1973): PO_2 Histogram of Three Dimensional Systems with Homogeneous and Inhomogeneous Microcirculation, a Digital computer Study. Oxygen Supply, edited by M. Kessler, D. Bruley, L. Clark, Jr., D. Lubbers, I. Silver, and J. Strauss, pp. 18-24. Urban & Schwarzenberg, Munchen.
36. Mochizuki, Masaji (1975): Graphical Analysis of Oxygenation and Co-Combination Rates of the Red Cells in the Lung. Hirokawa Publishing Company, Inc., Tokyo.
37. Pearson. (1905): The Problem of the Random Walk. Nature. 77:294.
38. Rayleigh, L. (1905): The Problem of the Random Walk. Nature 72:123.
39. Reneau, D. D., Slack, T. L., Bruley, D. F., Bicher, H. I., Knisely, J. H. (1973): A Systems Analysis of Oxygen and Glucose Transport in the Human Brain Under Conditions of Countercurrent Capillary Blood Flow. Bibl. Anat. 11:520-525.
40. Uhlenbeck, G. E. and Orstein, L. S. (1930): On the Theory of Brownian Motion. Phys. Review. 36:823.
41. Yowell, E. C. (1949): A Monte Carlo Method of Solving LaPlace's Equation. Proceedings of a Seminar on Scientific Computation: IBM Corporation, pp. 87-91. New York.
42. Williford, C. W., Bruley, D. F., and Artigue, R. S. (1979): The Probabalistic Modeling of Oxygen Transport in Brain Tissue. Proceedings of the Xth World Conference for Microcirculation. Sardinia.
43. Wyman, C. E. and Kosten, M. D. (1971): Stochastic Green's Function Method for Calculating the Concentration Profile of a Chemically Reactive Species. Chemical Engineering Computing, November.
44. Wodick, R. (1973): Stochastic Versus Deterministic Models of Oxygen Transport in the Tissue. Advances in Experimental Medicine and Biology, 37B.
45. Smoluchowski, M. V. "Drei Vortage Uber Diffusion, Brownsche, Bewlgung Und Koagulation von Kolloidteichen," Physik Zeifs, 17, 557 (1916).

Mathematics of Microcirculation Phenomena,
edited by J. F. Gross and A. Popel.
Raven Press, New York © 1980.

Micro-Macroscopic Scaling

J. S. Lee

Division of Biomedical Engineering, University of Virginia, Charlottesville, Virginia 22908

INTRODUCTION

The indicator dilution technique is a powerful method to identify certain vascular dynamics of an organ. Injecting non-
permeable indicators such as tagged red blood cells, one could
compute from the dilution curves the blood flow through the organ and its vascular volume (1). The introduction of permeable
substance has been used to quantify its extraction by the organ
(2). These derived informations are defined here as macroscale
quantities characterizing the vascular dynamics.

As the indicator is transported by the blood through an organ;
some flows through the capillaries, the major exchange or extraction sites. Other is shunted through the thoroughfare channels.
At a bifurcation of the microvascular network, red blood cells
prefer to flow into the daughter branch having faster flow (3).
These events are of microscale. They control the characteristics
of the indicator dilution curve. Thus it will be desirable to
study the effect of these microscaling events on the macroscaling
dilution curve. Such an integration study may help the development of methods to extract more information from indicator
dilution technique on the microvascular function.

NONUNIFORM TRANSPORT OF INDICATOR IN MICROVASCULATURE

After a pulse injection of the indicator into the arterial end
of an organ, the dilution curve at the venous end shows a time
delay on the arrival of indicator, a rapid rise in its concentration and then a decay. This dilution curve normalized by the
amount of indicator is designated as the transport function. It
is the distribution function of the transversal or residence time
of the indicator (1). The broadening of the distribution function from the impulse input and hence the large variation in the

159

residence time is the result of the irregular nature of the
micro-vascular flow, the nonuniform velocity profile in the
microvessels, etc.

One approach to resolve the macroscale event into microscale
ones is to idealize each of the arterial, capillary, and venous
systems as single electric elements having certain transport
functions. These three elements are organized in serial. Its
total transport function is obtained by the convolution of individual ones (4). The appropriate form of the transport function for the capillary element has been studied by Taylor for
circular tube (5) and by Fung for pulmonary sheet (4). However,
there is a lack of knowledge on the transport function for the
arterial and venous system. It is noted that this three element
model assumes that the input to all capillaries are identical.

Such a network analysis has been used extensively to investi-
gate the pressure and flow distribution of cardiovascular system
and in irregular microvascular organization (6,7). Could one
adapt the irregular network analysis for the microscale simulation of indicator transport? To examine this question closely,
let us look at the flow in an arterial bifurcation. For
Poiseuille flow, the velocity is non-uniform. However, the
pressure is uniformly distributed across the cross-section of the
tube. With the presence of a bifurcation, one could still approximate the input pressure to the daughter branches as equal.

On the other hand, the nonuniform velocity profile in the tube
flow and the non-symmetric arrangement of the bifurcation may
cause a large deviation in the indicator flow to the daughter
branches. To illustrate this point, we sketched in Fig. 1 the
movement of indicator along the tube in dark color for an
indicator bolus injected at the entrance. For a slower flow to
the upper branch, the streamline dividing the flow to the daughter branches will be skewed upward from the centerline as shown
by the broken line. As one can see that the arrival of the
indicator to the upper branch will lag from that to the lower
one. This non-uniform distribution in the indicator input is

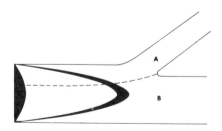

Figure 1.   Transport of indicator through a bifurcation flow.

amplified further as blood flows through many branchings in the arterial system. This amplification is illustrated by our observation of a wide distribution in the mean transit time for arterioles and venules of mesentery. Consequently, one essential requirement for a microscale analysis is to account for the non-uniform flow distribution throughout the whole microvascular network.

DISPERSION OF INDICATOR IN STREAMTUBE

The concept of residence time is centered on how long the indicator particle has resided in the vascular bed. This concept is capable to show, without detail knowledge about the microvascular flow, that the mean transit time is equal to the ratio of the vascular volume and the flow. However, the lack of direct association of the indicator particle with the functional unit of microvasculature makes this concept less adaptable for the integration of the microscale events.

One basic microvascular unit is the capillary. With the assumption that the filtration across the endothelium being much smaller than the blood flow and the blood is a homogenous continuum, we can consider the capillary as a streamtube. The extension of the streamtube upstream identifies its segment in the arterial system. Similar extension can be made for the venous segment. In this concept of streamtube, fluid flowing into the arterial end of the streamtube will stay in the streamtube until its exit at the venous end.

Taylor has examined the dispersion of indicator in straight, circular streamtube (5). Let d be the tube diameter, u the

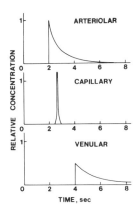

Figure 2. Transport function for the arterial (top), capillary (middle) and venous (bottom) segment of a streamtube.

average velocity of the fluid and D the diffusion coefficient of the indicator. Taylor showed that when du/D is very large, the nonuniform convective motion across the tube is the primary dispersion mechanism. The transport function is similar to the one shown in the top or bottom configuration of Figure 2. When du/D is small, the diffusion changes the dispersion character- istics to one of normal distribution as sketched in the middle. of Figure 2.

To bypass theoretical difficulty of constructing a streamtube in a complex microvascular flow and of computing the distribution of residence time, Nellis and Lee developed a microvascular di- lution technique to measure the dilution of indicator injected into the mesentery artery to the arterioles and the venules in the mesentery membrane (8). It was found that the experimental transport function for the arteriole, ha, could be reasonably simulated by

$$ha = 1(T - Ta) \ (Na/Ta) \ exp(- Na(\ T - Ta)/Ta) \qquad (1)$$

where·T is the time, Ta the (appearance) time for the indicator injected into the artery to show up first in the arteriole, 1(T) the unit step function, and Na the decay factor. As this trans- port function is comparable to that of Poiseuille flow with negligible diffusion, our measurements suggest that the dis- persion of indicator in the arterial segment of the streamtube is the result of non-uniform convection.

For a capillary flow velocity of 0.5mm/sec, a diameter of 8 µm, and a diffusion coefficient of $0.5x10^{-5}$ cm^2/sec, we have du/D = 0.4. The transport function for the capillary segment of the streamtube having this small dimensionless parameter is sketched in the middle of Fig. 2. In this theoretical consider- ation, Taylor assumed the flow to be Poiseuille (5). Because of the rapid diffusion in the radial direction of the infinitesmal capillary, most of the indicator remains concentrated in a small region as it flows along the capillary. This is in contrast to the wide dispersion seen in the arterial segment of the stream- tube. For the sake of simpler computation, this smaller dis- persion in the capillary is approximated by a pulse response described by the delta function:

$$hc = \delta \ (T - Tc) \qquad (2)$$

where Tc is the mean transit time for the indicator to flow through the capillary.

Because of the relative uniform concentration at the junction of the arterial and capillary segment, we can convolute Eq. 1 and 2 to find the transport function for the segment of streamtube in between the artery and the end of capillary:

$$ha.c = 1(T - Ta - Tc) \ Na/Ta \ exp(- Na(T - Ta - Tc)/Ta \ ) \quad (3)$$

A venule collects the flow from several streamtubes. The venular transport function is the sum of the individual functions of these streamtubes weighed by their flow. If the individual function is identical, the venular transport function should look like the one specified by Eq. 3. Our experimental observation of a much wider dispersion in the venule indicates a highly non-uniform flow distribution among the streamtubes.

The converging flow in the venous system makes it difficult to identify the dilution curve in the venous segment of the streamtube experimentally. As the Reynolds number of the vascular flow is small, the flow is governed by the Stokes equations which are linear. Thus the solution of a reversed flow can be obtained by changing the sign of the velocity. Consequently, the transport function for the venous segment, hv, of the streamtube will be similar to that of the arterial one:

$$hv = 1(T - Tv) \ Nv/Tv \ \exp(\ - \ Nv(T - Tv)/Tv) \qquad (4)$$

where Tv is the time between the indicator injected at the end of the capillary and the first appearance at the end of the venous segment. The effect of interstreamtube diffusion on hv will be discussed in the next section.

The transport function for the entire streamtube, hs, is the convolution integral of Eq. 3 and 4 which is given by

$$hs = 1(T^*) \ \frac{Na}{Ta} \frac{Nv}{Tv} \ / \ (\frac{Na}{Ta} - \frac{Nv}{Tv}) \ (\ \exp(- \frac{Na}{Ta}T^* \ )-\exp(\ - \frac{Nv}{Tv}T^*)) \ (5)$$

where $T^* = T - Ta - Tc - Tv$.

Our measurements on Ta show a wide range of 1.5 to 4.5 seconds. It could be simulated by the following lagged normal distribution

$$G(\theta) = (4\Pi \ a\theta)^{-\frac{1}{2}} \ \exp(\ -(1 - \theta)^2/(4a\theta) \ ) \qquad (6)$$

where $\theta = Ta/\overline{Ta} - b$ with a and b as constants and $\overline{Ta}$ as the mean appearance time for all arterial streamtubes. The decay factor, Na, is distributed over a much narrow range so we take Na = constant for all streamtubes. Because of experimental difficulty, Tc, Tv, and Nv have not been measured. It is possible that a slower flow or longer Ta in the arterial segment of a streamtube may associate with slower flow in its two downstream segments. In addition the flow in vein may be slower than the arterial ones. As a first attempt to integrate the dilution curves of individual streamtubes to the whole organ, we assume

$$Ta = Tc = Tv/2 \qquad (7)$$

The decay factor is affected by the flow configuration and not by the magnitude of the velocity. Consequently we take

$$Na = Nv = constant. \qquad (8)$$

With these simplifications, the transport function for the streamtube, Eq. 5, is simplified to

$$hs(T) = 1(T^*) \ Na/Ta \ (\ exp(\ -NaT^*/Ta) \ -exp(\ -NaT^*/(2Ta)\ )\ ) \quad (9)$$

where $T^* = T - 4Ta$. For $Ta = 2.5$ sec. and $Na = 1.4$, this transfer function is plotted as the broken line in Fig. 3. As one can see that the sudden increase in the transfer function of the arterial and venous streamtube at the appearance time is smoothened by the convolution. This curve is similar to the lagged normal distribution assumed by Bassingwaighte et. al. (8).

Based on the distribution function Eq. 6, the transport function for the whole organ, ho, is given by

$$ho(T) = \int_0^\infty G(Ta) \ hs(T,Ta) \ dTa/ \ \overline{Ta} \quad (10)$$

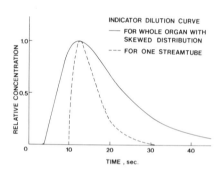

Figure 3. The computed transport function for an entire streamtube (broken line) and that of an organ derived from the summing of the transport function for all streamtubes.

The numerical integration for $\overline{Ta} = 2$ sec, $b = 0.25$ and $a = 0.2$ is shown as the solid line in Fig. 3. The wider distribution of transit time than that of the individual single streamtube reflects primarily the variation of indicator transport among the streamtubes. This form compares favorably with the dilution curve obtained from the kidney (2).

The present parallel pathway model differs from existing ones (10) in several aspects. Our model closely associates the pathway (or streamtube) with the functional unit of capillary. The transport function and distribution function used are derived from microvascular dilution experiments.

DIFFUSION AND MIXING OF INDICATOR AMONG STREAMTUBES

The concept of streamtube is applicable to the ideal flow of a homogeneous and continous fluid. In the capillary segment of the streamtube, non-permeable indicator is confined in the capillary by the endothelium. However, in the artery, the indicator is free to diffuse by molecular action to and to mix by the rotation of red blood cells with adjacent streamtubes.

To visualize this interstreamtube transport of the indicator, let us examine first in what form should the arterial segment of a streamtube be? Suppose it shapes like a circular tube. Since the cross-sectional area of the artery is smaller than the total cross-sectional area of all the downstream capillaries, the diameter of the arterial segment of the streamtube will be much smaller than the capillary one. Across such an infinitesimal dimension in the arterial flow, the velocity variation is so small that it will not be able to account for the large dispersion seen in the arterioles of the mesentery membrane (8). Thus the most likely configuration for the arterial segment of the streamtube is a ribbon structure having a large width to produce the needed variation in the convective velocity but a thin sheet to preserve a small cross-sectional area.

Take a point A in an arterial ribbon. We can find from the adjacent streamtube a point B which is separated from A by the thickness of the ribbon. The infinitesmal distance between these two points indicates a negligible velocity variation in the macroscopic, nonuniform arterial flow. Therefore the indicator injected in the entrance of the artery will reach both points almost at the same time. No significant concentration gradient of the indicator could be developed to induce net transport A and B. Thus, the arterial transport function is insignificantly affected by the small interstreamtube diffusion. This argument is supported by our experimental suggestion that the indicator transport from artery to arteriole is primarily convective.

Among the several streamtubes of a venule, the variation in transit time is large. Large concentration gradient could be developed between point A and B in these streamtubes to induce a diffusion or mixing, say, from A to B. Because of the infinitesmal distance between A and B, the fluid particle in A and B will convect to the venous outlet at the same instant. Thus, the net flux of indicator from A to B will be carried by the fluid particle in B to the outlet as if the indicator were carried by the fluid particle at A. In other words, the interstreamtube transport may alter significantly the transport function of an individual streamtube. When the effects are summed over all the streamtubes, the alteration to the overall transport function becomes minimal.

If this interstreamtube diffusion is important, the overall transport function should be affected by the diffusion coefficient. Similar transport found for widely different molecules (sodium ion and T 1824) and red blood cells through the pulmonary vasculature may be an indirect evidence to support our previous conclusion on interstreamtube diffusion (11, 12).

ROLE OF SHUNT FLOW IN INDICATOR DISPERSION

To account for the role of shunt flow in indicator dispersion, one forms a set of streamtubes generated from the thoroughfare channels. Although there is no direct microvascular measurement on what fraction the shunt flow is, the measurement of hematocrit in the capillaries may be used to evaluate the shunt flow. Let Q_c be the total flow through the streamtubes formed by the capillaries and Q_s be those from the thoroughfare channels. Then the conservation of red blood cells require that:

$$(Q_c + Q_s)\ Ha = Q_c\ Hc + Q_s\ Hs \qquad (11)$$

where H is the collecting hematocrit with the subscript a,c,s, indicating the artery, the capillary and the shunt respectively. Let Δ be the fraction of shunt flow $(= Q_s/Q_c + Q_s))$. The equation above is simplified to:

$$\Delta\ Hs + (1-\Delta)\ Hc = Ha \qquad (12)$$

For a given fraction of shunt flow, Eq. 12 establishes the one-to-one relationship between the capillary hematocrit and that of shunt flow. Their relations for a range of Δ are plotted in Figure 4.

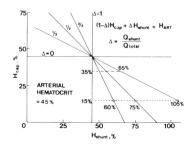

Figure 4.   The relation between the capillary and shunt hematocrit as a function of fractional shunt flow (Δ).

Many investigators have found that the hematocrit in capillary is in the range of 8 to 15% (13,14). If the shunt flow is one third of the total flow, we find that the shunt hematocrit has to be 105% in order to balance a 15% hematocrit in the capillary. On the other hand, if we consider that the shunt hematocrit can at most be 60%, then the relation shown in Figure 4 suggests that the shunt flow is 2/3 of the total flow. As the capillary hematocrit should be converted to feed hematocrit to account for the Fahreaus effect, a slight modification of the estimation on the shunt flow is expected.

In contrast to the streamtube of the capillary, the indicator in the shunted ones should move faster along the thoroughfare channel and appear early in the vein. For a permeable substance passing through the shunting streamtube, it should experience less extraction. One of the mechanisms proposed to explain the hematocrit difference among microvessels is the preference of red blood cells to stay in daughter branch with faster flow. This branch may possibly be the thoroughfare channel. Thus if the shunt flow is significant in micro-scale, the shunted indicator (especially the red blood cells) should show up in the dilution curve (the macro-scale) early and exhibit less extraction. This suggestion is not supported by macroscale experiments. Crone found that the indicator extraction in kidney is constant for the first few seconds after the appearance of the indicator in the vein (2). After appropriate correction on the transport of red blood cells and T 1824, Dow found only a slight lead by the red blood cells (12). Further study along the concept of streamtube may help us to identify this conflicting role of shunt flow implied by micro-scale hematocrit measurement and macro-scale dilution curve.

SUMMARY

The concept of streamtube allows us to examine the indicator transport in an organ in the perspective of microscale. The experimental and theoretical investigations suggest various modes of indicator transport along a streamtube. The irregular flow distribution among streamtubes is one major factor in widening the transport function of the whole organ. This concept to associate the transport function with the functional unit of the microvasculature may be useful for better understanding of the indicator dilution technique and for the determination of shunt flow in organs.

REFERENCES

1. Zierler, K. L. (1964): Circulation times and the theory of indicator dilution methods for determining flood flow and volume. In Handbook of Physiology Sec. II, Circ. vol. 1, Edited by W. F. Hamilton and D. Dow, Am. Physiol. Soc., p. 585-615.

2. Crone, C. (1963): The permeability of capillaires in various organs as determined by use of the indicator-diffusion method. Acta. Physiol. Scand. 58: 292-305.

3. Johnson, P. C. (1971): Red cell separation in the mesenteric capillary network, J. Appl. Physiol., 221: 99-104.

4. Fung, Y.C., and Sobin, S. S. (1972) pulmonary alveolar blood flow, Circ. Res, 30: 470-488.

5. Taylor, G. (1953): Dispersion of soluble matter in solvent flowing slowly through a tube. Proc. Royal. Soc. London, Ser. A., 219: 186-203.

6. Lipowsky, H. H., and Zweifach, B. W. (1974): Network analysis of microcirculation of cat mesentery. Microvas. Res., 7:73-83.

7. Lee, J. S. and Nellis, S. H., (1974): Modeling study on the distribution of flow and volume in the microcirculation of cat mesentery. Ann. Biomed. Eng. 2: 206-216.

8. Nellis, S. H., Lee, J. S. (1974): Dispersion of indicator measured from microvessels of cat mesentery, Circ. Res. 35: 580-591.

9. Bassingthwaighte, J. B., Ackerman, F. H., and Wood, E. H. (1966): Application of the lagged normal density curve as a model for arterial dilution curves. Circ. Res., 18: 398-415.

10. Bassingthwaighte, J. B. (1970): Blood flow and diffusion through mammalian organs, Science, 167: 1347-1353.

11. Chinard, F. P., and Enns. T., (1954): Transcapillary pulmonary exchange of water in the dog, Am. J. Physiol., 178: 192-202.

12. Dow, P., Hahn, P. F., and Hamilton, W. F. (1946): The simultaneous transport of T-1824 and radioactive red blood cells through the heart and lungs, Am. J. Physics., 147: 493-499.

13. Schmid-Schonbein, G. W., and Zweifach, B. W. (1975): RBC velocity profiles in arterioles and venules of the rabbit omentum. Microvas. Res., 10: 153-164.

14. Lipowsky, H. H., and Zweifach, B. W. (1977): Methods for the simultaneous measurement of pressure differentials and flow in a single unbranched vessel of the microcirculation for rheological studies. Microvas. Res., 14: 345-361.

ACKNOWLEDGEMENT

This work is supported by Grant HL 23769 and a Research Career Development Award K04 HL 00004 from the National Heart, Lung, and Blood Institute.

Subject Index

Absorption, fluid, in intestinal
  muscle, 53–55
Arteriolar network
  diverging structure of, 68–71
  transit times in, 72
Arteriolar vessel
  diverging structure of, 68
  and tissue, oxygen exchange,
    73–74
Arteriole(s)
  characteristics of, 7
  dimensionless volumetric flow
    rate at, 71
  transport function for, 162
Axisymmetric cases, flow mechanics
    of, 17–37

Basement membrane in capillaries
  characteristics and composition
    of, 8
  rigidity of, 10
  thickness of, 9–11
Bending strain energy, 31
Blake and Gross densitometric
    (BGD) microocclusion tech-
    nique, 59–60
Blood flow, vascular elasticity and, 1
Blood vessels
  arterioles, 7
  capillaries, 7–11
  elasticity of, 1, 2–7
    inversion of stress-strain
      relationship, 5–7
Brain, oxygen transport in, 133–156;
    see also Oxygen transport in
    brain microcirculation
Brownian motion, 135–136

Capillary(ies), 7–11
  characteristics of, 7–9
  dispersion of indicator in, 162

geometry of, 42–43
mesentery, 9–10
parallel, as model, 79–80
transcapillary fluid exchange
  theory and, 51–53
"tunnel in gel" concept and, 8,
  9–11
Capillary and shunt hematocrit, 166
Capillary permeability determination, 55–60
Capillary-tissue exchange theory,
  93–96
Capillary-tissue oxygen exchange,
  77–83
Conductivity, hydraulic, see
  Hydraulic conductivity
Cones, rigid truncated, pressures of,
  29
Connective tissue, capillary, 8, 9–11
Convection and diffusion problems,
  89–107
  linear steady, 101–104
  non-linear steady, 96–101
  unsteady periodic, 104–106
Convective and diffusive transport,
  63–83
  capillary-tissue oxygen exchange
    in, 77–83
  flow and pressure distribution
    in, 64–73
  precapillary oxygen losses in,
    73–77
Cubic lattice model, 78
Cylindrical tubes, flow in, 21–27

Darcy's law, 92
Diameter ratios and viscosities and
    pressure drops, 32, 33, 35
Diffusion
  in extravascular space, 89–107